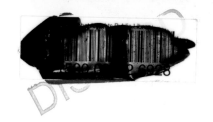
200
Surefire Ways to
Eat Well & Feel Better

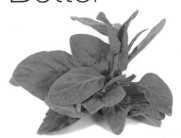

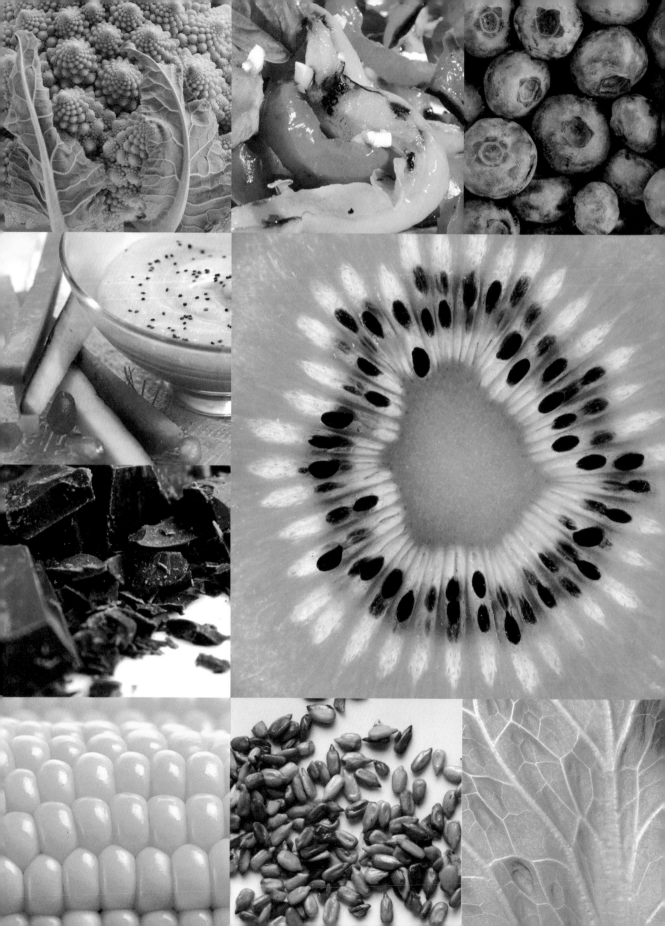

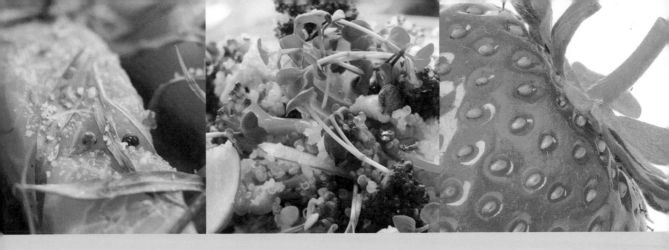

200

Surefire Ways to
Eat Well & Feel Better

Dr. Judith Rodriguez

Fair Winds Press
100 Cummings Center, Suite 406L
Beverly, MA 01915

fairwindspress.com • quarryspoon.com

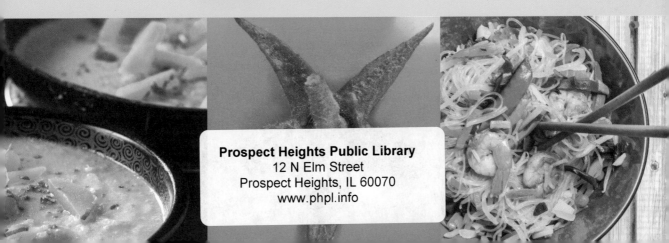

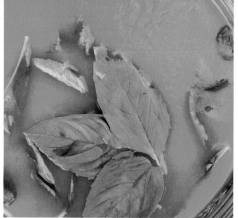
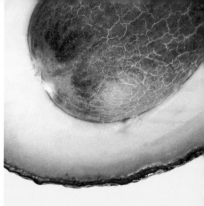

A QUARTO BOOK
Copyright © 2014 Quarto Inc.

First published in the USA in 2014 by
Fair Winds Press, a member of
Quarto Publishing Group USA Inc.
100 Cummings Center
Suite 406-L
Beverly, MA 01915-6101
www.fairwindspress.com

Visit www.bodymindbeautyhealth.com.
It's your personal guide to a happy, healthy,
and extraordinary life!

ISBN: 978-1-59233-653-1

Digital edition published in 2014
eISBN: 978-1-62788-221-7

Library of Congress Cataloging-in-Publication
Data available

Conceived, designed, and produced by
Quarto Publishing plc
The Old Brewery, 6 Blundell Street
London N7 9BH

QUAR.FTTE

Senior editor: **Katie Crous**
Copy editor: **Ruth Patrick**
Proofreader: **Liz Jones**
Designer: **Karin Skånberg**
Design assistant: **Martina Calvio**
Photographer: **Simon Pask**
Illustrator: **Justin Gabbard**
Picture researcher: **Sarah Bell**
Art director: **Caroline Guest**
Creative director: **Moira Clinch**
Publisher: **Paul Carslake**

Color separation in Hong Kong by Cypress
Colors (HK) Ltd
Printed in China by 1010 Printing International Ltd

10 9 8 7 6 5 4 3 2 1

The information in this book is for educational
purposes only. It is not intended to replace the
advice of a physician or medical practitioner.
Please see your health care provider before
beginning any new health program.

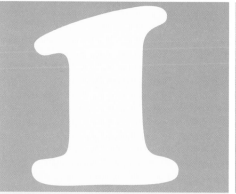

Contents

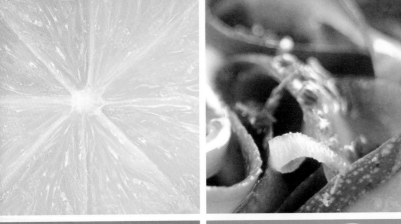
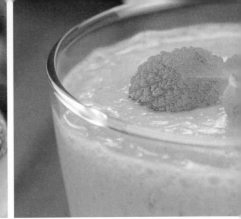

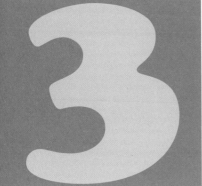

3 4 5

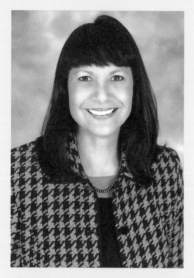

Eating smart, losing weight, and keeping the weight off does not have to be difficult. With some personalized and convenient changes to your diet, physical activity, and lifestyle, you will soon be feeling good and living better.

This book is organized into five sections, each of which addresses an aspect of daily life: At home, Shopping, Restaurants and parties, Diets and eating plans, and Special health concerns. As a step in the right direction, try to adopt a few tips from each of the sections. Once those tips have become a healthy habit, adopt a few more. If you select a tip and find it is not working, come back to the book and look for some others to try instead. Pick the tips you think are relevant and applicable to you.

When trying to implement food, physical activity, and lifestyle changes you can easily become overwhelmed. But the research shows that taking small steps can help you succeed in your attempts. Being healthy is achievable if you take an honest look at all aspects of your lifestyle, know what and how to change, and stay motivated. This book will help you do all of these things.

Judith C. Rodriguez
Ph.D., R.D.N., L.D./N., F.A.D.A.
Chairperson and Professor, Department of Nutrition and Dietetics, Brooks College of Health, Florida

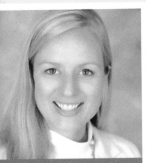

Jenna Braddock, M.S.H., R.D.N., C.S.S.D., is an Instructor at the University of North Florida and a Nutrition Consultant.
• Start the party right—appetizers 82 • Enjoy the party—right! Main dishes 84–85 • Detox diets 96–97 • Fueling the athlete 130–131

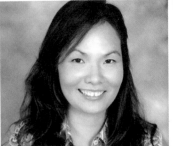

Kate Chang, M.S., R.D.N., is an Adjunct Instructor at the University of North Florida and a Nutrition Consultant.
• Dinner: The healthy option 30–33
• Shopping for snacks 60–61
• Healthy dining at restaurants: Japanese cuisine 77

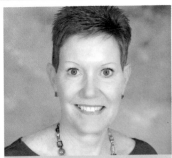

Catherine Christie, Ph.D., R.D.N., is Associate Dean at the University of North Florida.
• Cooking for many 22–25 • Calories and serving sizes 62–63 • Healthy dining at restaurants: Italian cuisine 76 • Nutrigenomics: What's in it for you? 94–95 • The Paleo diet 106–107 • Food and mood 132–133

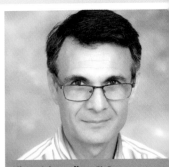

Alireza Jahan-mihan, Ph.D., R.D.N., is an Assistant Professor at the University of North Florida.
• Aging well 122–123
• Nutrition for men 126–127

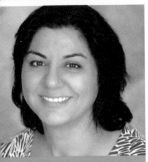

Shahla Khan, Ph.D., is an Adjunct Instructor at the University of North Florida and Jacksonville University.
• Getting and staying active 36–41

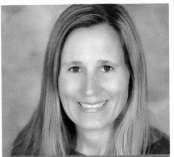

Corinne Labyak, Ph.D., R.D.N., is an Assistant Professor at the University of North Florida.
• High blood pressure 116–117
• Nutrition for children 128–129

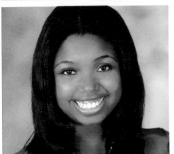

Jamisha Laster, M.S., R.D.N., is an Adjunct Instructor at the University of North Florida and a Senior Public Health Nutritionist.
• Healthy dining at restaurants: Soul food 74

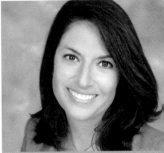

Alexia Lewis, M.S., R.D.N., is a Wellness Dietitian at the University of North Florida and a Nutrition Consultant.
• Snacks: Boosting your nutrition 34–35 • The raw food diet 100–101 • The vegan diet 102–103 • The DASH diet 104–105 • Heart disease 118–119 • Gluten sensitivity 136–137

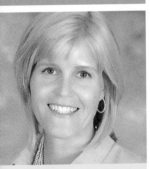

Jen Ross, M.S.H., R.D.N., is an Instructor at the University of North Florida and a Nutrition Consultant.
• Cooking and baking made easy 14–17
• Cooking for one 18–21

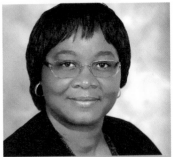

Claudia Sealey-Potts, Ph.D., R.D.N., is an Assistant Professor at the University of North Florida.
• Healthy dining at restaurants: Chinese cuisine 75
• Be ingredient savvy 64–65
• Diabetes 114–115

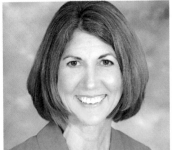

Jackie Shank, M.S., R.D.N., is an Instructor at the University of North Florida.
• Nutrition for women 124–125
• Food allergies 134–135

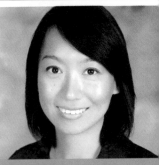

Zhiping Yu, Ph.D., R.D.N., is an Assistant Professor at the University of North Florida.
• Shopping for vegetables 48–49
• Shopping for fruit 50–51
• End the party right—sweets 83
• Enjoy the party—right! Main dishes 84–85 • Healthy drinking practices 86–87

About this book

The five chapters in this book each address a key aspect of eating well—whether it's in your home or out and about, or adopting specific dietary changes in order to meet your specific needs and desires for a healthier lifestyle.

Chapters 2 and 3: Out and about: Shopping, pages 42–67; Restaurants and parties, pages 68–87

In Chapter 2 you'll find plenty of tips for shopping for all food types, comparing calories and serving sizes, understanding the ingredients on labels, and buying snacks. Then be guided through the maze of fast-food menus and popular ethnic dishes available at restaurants. Finally, whether hosting or attending, parties are often a time when you may find it difficult to make healthy choices and this section can help you through those dilemmas.

Chapter 1: At home, pages 10–41

Perhaps the easiest—and most important—place to make a start is in your own home. This chapter looks at how you can make the most of your time in the kitchen, preparing and cooking the right kind of meals, and staying active without even leaving your front door.

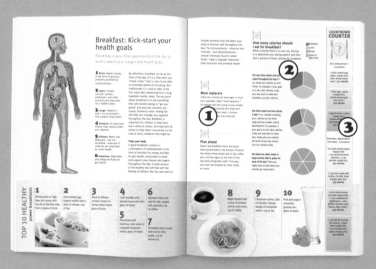

1 Hints and tips
Concise snippets of information and advice for making changes toward a healthier lifestyle.

2 Reference charts
Easy-to-digest charts show important facts and figures.

3 Countdown counters
Comparative lists of foods in ascending order of calories or descending order of specific nutrients (check the individual Counter heading). Calories and nutritional values are an indication only; both will vary greatly depending on how the food is made and the serving size.

Chapter 4: Diets and eating plans, pages 88–109

Discover the rationale behind popular diets and the strength of the science behind them. Assess the pros and cons and take a look at some sample menus before you decide on the best option for you.

Chapter 5: Special health concerns, pages 110–137

Common chronic diseases, such as diabetes, and food allergies and/or sensitivities can be better managed with appropriate dietary changes. Women, men, children, the elderly, and athletes all have specific needs and this section will help you identify issues and gain the maximum benefit from food.

About this book 9

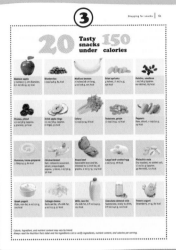
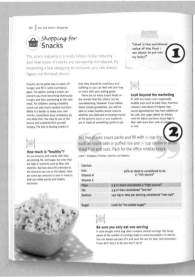

1 Fridge magnet mantras
Motivating boosts to write down and place in a prominent location.

2 Expert quotes
Additional insider advice from professionals in the field of nutrition.

3 Top foods
At-a-glance illustrated lists of the best foods available for your dietary needs.

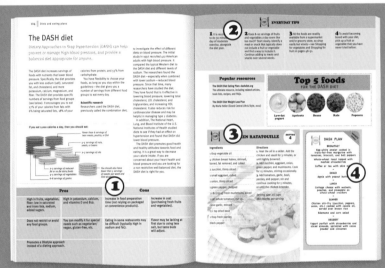

1 Pros and cons
Weigh up the positives and the negatives of each diet.

2 Everyday tips
Small changes you can make to daily life to help you follow each diet.

3 Healthy recipes
Quick and easy recipes—including ingredients and nutritional details—that you can try at home.

4 Sample menus
Guides to the type of meals you can expect to eat when following a specific eating plan.

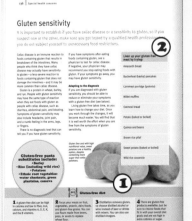
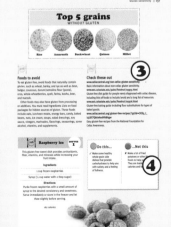

1 Specific guidelines
Follow the advice and manage your health easily and effectively.

2 Meal ideas
Lists of healthy meal enhancers and ingredient substitutions provide plenty of inspiration for mealtimes.

3 Check these out
Websites offering additional information for further reading.

4 Do this/Not this
Identify unhealthy behavioral practices and find alternatives for smarter choices.

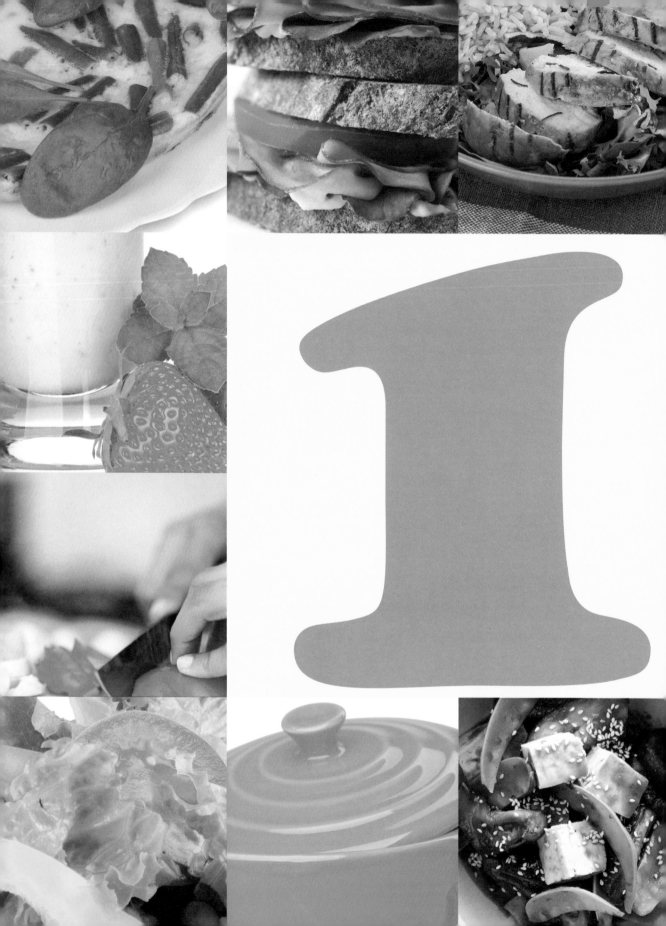

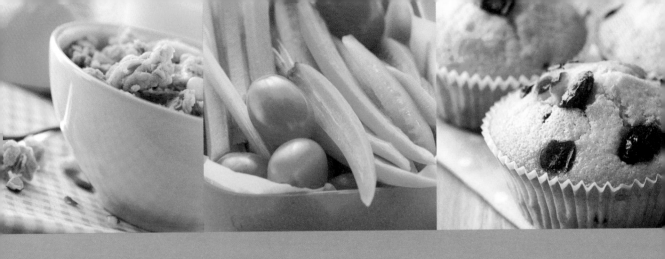

At home

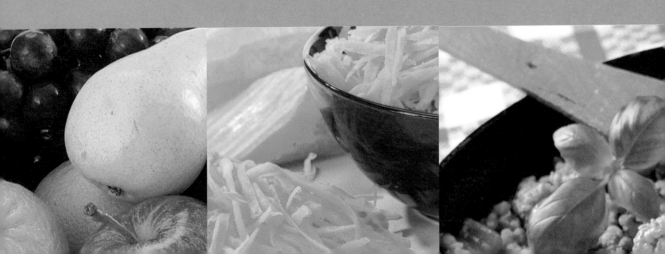

A healthy life starts at home

What you learned when growing up at home most likely formed the foundation of what you currently do, whether it's managing your weight, life, or work.

Home was your first school. This is where you learned how to interact with others and developed food and physical activity habits. You learned basic life management skills, such as shopping, cooking, and how to manage stress and emotions through dialogue and relationships. A home is also where you may have learned behaviors that have become problematic and hard to correct. These may include using food as an emotional outlet when angry or upset, using food to demonstrate love, eating excessively during specific holidays or celebrations, or watching television for many hours at a time. To create a healthier lifestyle, begin with small changes at home and turn them into lifelong benefits you can take with you anywhere you go.

Your personality, lifestyle, and values are reflected in your home, particularly the kitchen and activity niches. What do your home and color schemes say about your lifestyle? Key to making lifestyle improvements that support weight loss or maintenance is to work not only on your personal behaviors, but also to create a home environment that supports the goals you are trying to achieve.

Check these out

www.caloriesecrets.net
10 tips on how to develop healthy eating habits.
www.healthcastle.com/healthy_kitchen_staple.shtml
Kitchen staples for healthy family meals.
www.styleathome.com/kitchen-and-bath/kitchen
Eight steps to designing a healthy kitchen.

Four steps to create a supportive home environment

1 Use fruits as a table centerpiece and healthy snack option.

2 Place exercise motivators in key positions, such as a jump rope in the garage or weights by the sofa.

3 Create a quiet space in which to relax, such as a comfy chair in the bedroom or rocker on the patio.

4 Keep a scale by the shower. Use it twice weekly.

Get active in the home

Get a pedometer and commit to walking a specific number of steps in the home, say 2,000. Walk around the sofa, step in place, walk up and down the stairs, or run after the dog (or kids). Do it every day and make it fun.

Do this...

✓ Encourage family members to eat until almost but not overly full.

✓ Focus on pleasant conversation and interactions during mealtimes rather than watching TV.

...Not this

✗ Use food to compensate for, or protect against, sad feelings.

✗ Use highly sweetened or fatty foods as a reward or tease for promoting good behaviors in children.

Every home needs one
Fill your fruit bowl with fruit of different colors and shapes for attractiveness, choice, and nutrient variety.

Before eating that food, ask yourself: "Am I really hungry?"

Big on energy, bananas also have potassium, important in heart health, and are the original prepackaged snack.

Pears are packed with antioxidants, fiber, and flavor!

Ideal for grazing, grapes contain resveratrol, an antioxidant that helps fight cancer and heart disease.

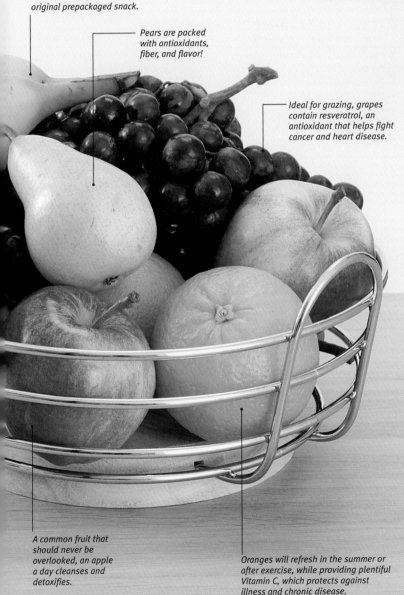

A common fruit that should never be overlooked, an apple a day cleanses and detoxifies.

Oranges will refresh in the summer or after exercise, while providing plentiful Vitamin C, which protects against illness and chronic disease.

(4)

Remodel your home

Make each room in your home a welcome supporter of your goals. Go to each room and assess the environment. Identify small, cost-free, or inexpensive changes you can make.

Den or sitting room: Are there any small dishes containing high-calorie snacks? Replace them with decorative stones or pinecones from your backyard.

Exercise room or corner: Place your favorite fitness equipment in a common and popular area to encourage you to use it. Decorate with green accents or walls to give you a feeling of greenery and the outdoors, and decrease the perception of exertion.

Kitchen: Do you have high-fat cream-based dressings or high-sodium/salt condiments in your pantry? Replace them with healthier substitutes such as olive oil, flavored vinegars, and garlic powder. Avoid using the color red on your walls, which may stimulate the appetite, but instead try using smaller red dishes for snack plates. That "red" may help signal "stop."

Shower: Relax with some lavender-, chamomile-, or bergamot-scented soaps if you shower at night. Use citrus-, jasmine-, or peppermint-scented soaps to help you wake up if you shower in the morning.

Bedroom: Do you have a TV? Replace it with a music system and play some soothing sleep or sea sounds. Use cool blue colors or light pastel shades of blue, gray, or green on your walls.

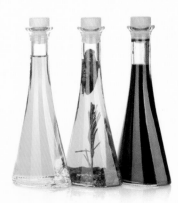

Cooking and baking made easy

Enjoy healthy cooking and eating at home while saving time and calories.

Preparing delicious and healthy foods at home doesn't have to be boring or time consuming. There are some basic steps you can take to help make cooking at home easy and successful.

Think ahead

Think about your family's meal preferences, budget, and time. It's important to work around these to make mealtimes more successful and less stressful. Meal planning is an important tool. Take a look at your weekly schedule and plan accordingly. If you know that one night is particularly hectic, plan for leftovers or a quick meal that night. Gather some familiar recipes plus some new ones to try and choose recipes that are within your cooking level and don't require equipment or time that you don't have. Cookbooks, websites, and blogs are great resources for recipe ideas and meal planning.

Broaden your skill set

Online videos are useful for learning new techniques and kitchen skills. If you want to advance your kitchen skills, consider taking a cooking class at a local college. The more flexible you can be with the ingredients you can cook and the methods you can use in the kitchen, the more likely you are to stick with healthy changes.

Shop smart and stock your pantry

Make a list of staples to always have on hand to save time and money at the grocery store. If you're trying to cut down on calories, be sure to have some low-sodium stock, vegetables, herbs, spices, and whole grains on hand. Acknowledge which ingredients you're more likely to use versus unfamiliar or expensive items. For example, if you find that you're constantly throwing out fresh produce, try buying more frozen vegetables and working some of the fresh in as you have time. See Chapter 2 for more advice on shopping for health.

Preparation is key

Many people are hesitant to cook because they're tired and don't want to think about putting something together after a long day at work. A little time prepping on the weekend can save you a lot of time and calories (not to mention money) during the week. Take an hour or two to plan your meals and pre-prep ingredients for the week. Go ahead and chop the vegetables for the stir-fry, or make the green salad. Put the meat in the refrigerator to defrost. Prepare and store any marinade.

You can't always tell by looking or smelling whether a food has gone bad, so to be safe, always use the mantra "when in doubt, throw it out."

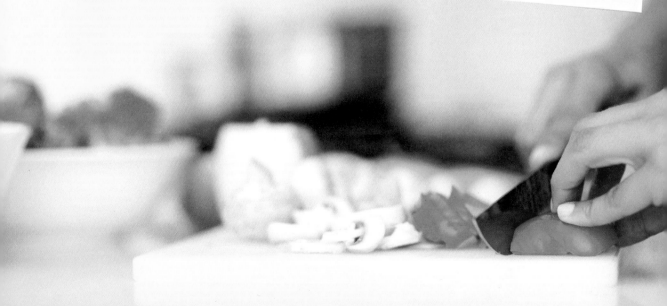

Maximizing nutrients

The chart on the right gives the optimum cooking times for popular vegetables. Use it as a guide, as times will vary by size, quantity, type of cut, and temperature cooked at.

Food safety first

Food safety is an important consideration when cooking at home.

• **Store raw meats, poultry, and seafood separate from other foods in the refrigerator,** preferably on the bottom shelf to keep any juices from dripping onto other items. Or simply freeze these foods if you don't plan on using them within a few days. Avoid cross-contamination and use separate utensils and cutting boards for produce, meat/poultry, seafood, and eggs.

• **Thaw your frozen meat and poultry in the refrigerator, in a bowl of cold water, or in the microwave (carefully following instructions for your model).** Do not thaw frozen foods out on the counter at room temperature—unless the packet instructions specify this method—because the food may become contaminated.

• **If storing leftovers, cool as quickly as possible and put in the refrigerator no more than two hours after cooking.** Most leftovers can be safely kept in the refrigerator for two to three days.

VEGETABLE	STEAM (MINUTES)	BOIL (MINUTES)	MICROWAVE (MINUTES)	BLANCH (MINUTES)	BAKE/ ROAST (MINUTES)
Artichoke, whole	30–40	30–45	5–7	n/a	n/a
Asparagus	8–10	5–10	4–6	2–3	8–10
Beans, green	5–15	10–20	6–12	4–5	n/a
Beets	40–60	30–60	14–18	n/a	60
Broccoli, spears	8–12	5–10	6–7	3–4	15–20
Brussels sprouts	6–12	5–10	7–8	4–5	30–40
Cabbage, wedges	6–9	10–15	10–12	n/a	20–25
Carrots, sliced	4–5	5–10	4–7	3–4	20
Cauliflower, florets	6–10	5–8	3–4	3–4	20–25
Corn, on cob	6–10	4–7	3–4	3–4	30
Eggplant, diced	15–20	10–20	7–10	3–4	10–15
Kale	4–7	5–10	3–6	4–5	20–25
Mushrooms	4–5	3–4	3–4	3–5	20–35
Onions, whole	25–40	15–20	6–10	4	50–60
Parsnips, whole	30–35	15–25	7–8	3–4	45–60
Peas, green	5–15	10–15	5–7	1–2	60
Peppers, bell	2–4	4–5	2–4	2–3	40
Potatoes, whole	30–45	30–40	6–8	3–5	40–60
Potatoes, cut	30–35	20–30	5–7	3–5	25–30
Spinach	6–12	3–10	3–7	2–3	25–30
Squash, sliced	30–40	20–25	6–7	3	40–50
Tomatoes	10	5–15	4–6	1–2	20–30
Turnips, diced	20–25	15–20	12–14	2–3	30–45
Zucchini, sliced	5–10	5–10	3–6	2–3	20–30

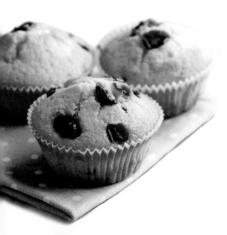

Enhancing baked goods

If you like baked goods but don't like the extra calories, consider baking at home. You can start with a prepackaged mix and reduce the calories by substituting a fruit purée such as applesauce for the oil.

Also consider ways to boost the nutrition in your baked goods. Adding fresh or frozen fruit, using whole-grain flours, flaxseeds, and reducing the fat are all easy ways to increase the nutrition without compromising the flavor.

Additionally, many baked goods can easily be frozen and reheated for later consumption. Replace store-bought frozen items with homemade muffins, pancakes, waffles, and breads as these items are all easy to make at home and freeze well.

Nutritional information

Vegetables are a great, easy way to fill up on nutrients. Most vegetables are low in fat and calories, but high in nutrients and fiber, which help you stay full for longer. Try to vary your vegetables and eat a range of colors. The different colors signify different phytonutrients, powerful compounds that help fight disease. Cook your vegetables in as little water as possible for the shortest amount of time possible to retain those important nutrients.

The data in this chart represents a ½ cup of cooked vegetables unless otherwise noted. Percentages of daily values (DV) are based on a 2,000-calorie diet.

Vegetable	Calories	Total Fat (g)	Sodium (mg)	Carbohydrates (g)	Fiber (g)	Sugar (g)	Protein (g)	% DV Vitamin A	% DV Vitamin C	% DV Iron	% DV Calcium
Artichoke, medium	60	1	120	13	6	1	4	0	25	9	6
Asparagus	20	0	12	3.5	1.5	1	2	18	12	5	2
Beans, green	18	0	16	4	1.5	0	1	8	7	6	3
Beets	37	0	65	8.5	1.5	6.5	1	1	5	4	1
Broccoli	27	0	32	5.5	2.5	1	2	24	84	3	3
Brussels sprouts	28	0	16	5.5	2	1	2	12	81	5	3
Cabbage	17	0	6	4	1	2	1	1	47	1	4
Carrots	27	0	45	6	2	2	0.5	266	5	1	2
Cauliflower	14	0	9	2.5	1	1	1	0	46	1	1
Corn on cob, medium	111	1	17	25	2.5	4	3	0	11	3	0
Eggplant	20	0	2	5	3	2	1	0	3	1	1
Kale	33	0	29	7	1	1.5	2	206	134	6	9
Mushrooms	23	0	5	4	1	1	2	0	0	2	2
Onions	64	0	6	15	3	7	2	0	20	2	4
Parsnips	100	0	13	24	7	6	2	0	38	4	5
Peas	117	1	7	21	7	8	8	22	97	12	4
Peppers, bell	30	0	4	7	3	4	1	11	200	3	1
Potatoes	164	0	13	39	5	2	4	0	70	9	3
Spinach	7	0	24	1	1	0	1	56	14	5	3
Squash	18	0	2	4	1	2	1	5	32	2	2
Tomatoes	32	0	9	7	2	5	2	30	38	3	2
Turnips	36	0	87	8	2	5	1	0	46	2	4
Zucchini	20	0	12	4	1	2	2	5	35	2	2

TOP 10 Recipe substitutions

1 **Applesauce** or other fruit purée is a great substitute for oil in baked goods, at a one-to-one ratio.

2 **Use low-sodium broth** or stock instead of oil when sautéing to decrease fat and calories.

3 **Whole-wheat flour** can be used to substitute half of the all-purpose flour in baked goods to increase nutrients, including fiber.

4 **Substitute yogurt** for sour cream as a condiment or for oil in baking.

5 **Use herbs and spices** instead of added salt as a flavor booster.

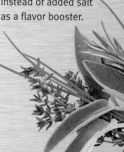

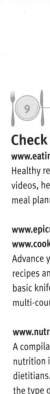

Check these out

www.eatingwell.com
Healthy recipes and features such as videos, healthy eating information, and meal planning tools.

www.epicurious.com and **www.cookinglight.com**
Advance your kitchen skills with recipes and videos that range from basic knife skills to preparing a multi-course dinner.

www.nutritionblognetwork.com
A compilation of blogs, with trusted nutrition information by registered dietitians. Search its directory to find the type of blog you're looking for. Categories include diabetes, family nutrition, vegetarian, weight management, and many more.

The perfect pan

A good non-stick skillet is easy to clean and an essential tool to make cooking easy. Choose a pan with high enough sides so that you can stir ingredients around easily. Start with some meat and some vegetables and grains for an easy one-pan weeknight meal.

For a fuller tummy, add vegetables to other foods.

• Add extra veggies to soups, casseroles, pasta dishes, and even baked goods.

• Add shredded carrots and zucchini to muffins and breads.

• Make vegetable purées ahead of time and freeze in ice-cube trays.

• Add the purées to pasta dishes and baked goods (be sure the vegetable is similar in color to the main dish).

6
Replace up to 50% of the fat in baked goods with cooked bean purées, and use puréed black beans in brownies and puréed white beans in cookies.

7
Use cooking spray instead of butter or shortening to prevent sticking.

8
Substitute two egg whites for one egg or use one tablespoon of ground flaxseed mixed with three tablespoons of water to replace one egg in a recipe to boost nutrition.

9
Use extra-lean ground beef or ground turkey/ chicken breast without skin for recipes that call for ground beef.

10
Reduce up to half of the amount of sugar called for in most recipes without compromising taste or texture.

Cooking for one

Save money and calories while preparing nutritious and delicious meals for one at home.

Cooking for one doesn't have to be boring or require complicated math to scale down recipes designed to serve four or more people. In fact, cooking for one can be very gratifying, and it allows you to explore and experiment with different flavors you may not otherwise try when cooking for others.

You can apply most of the same basic preparation as for Cooking for many (see pages 22–25). The main rules apply:
• Preparation is key and meal planning will save you valuable time during the week.
• Pay close attention to your recipes to avoid those ingredients you won't use often.
• Invest in some cookbooks or find websites and blogs that feature recipes for one.

Shopping for one can be costly, especially if you end up wasting food. Plan your meals (breakfast, lunch, dinner, and snacks) for the week. This will help ensure that you are eating a variety of foods. It will help you save money because you won't buy too much food that will end up spoiling, and it will make eating out less tempting. From your weekly menu, make a grocery list of only the foods that you will need for the meals. Write the list down and take it with you to the store. Sticking to your list will prevent the impulse to overbuy.

Simple and hearty vegetable soup

Stock up on a versatile soup like this one. Mix and match the ingredients with the vegetables and spices you have on hand. Freeze leftovers in single-serve containers for a quick lunch or evening meal.

8 servings

Ingredients
• 1 tbsp olive oil
• 1 onion, diced
• 3 carrots, diced
• 3 cloves garlic, minced
• 1 stalk celery, diced
• 1 cup shredded cabbage
• 1–2 bay leaves
• 1 cup chopped asparagus
• 1 lb new potatoes, diced
• 4 cups low-sodium vegetable broth

Directions

1. Heat the olive oil in a large pan. Add the onion, stir occasionally, and cook until translucent, about 5 minutes.

2. Add the carrots and garlic and cook for about 5 minutes or until garlic is fragrant. Add the celery, cabbage, and bay leaves and cook for another 5 minutes.

3. Add the asparagus, potatoes, and broth. Bring to a boil, then simmer uncovered for about 20–25 minutes or until the potatoes are soft enough to pierce with a fork. Season with salt (go easy!) and pepper to taste.

90 calories per serving

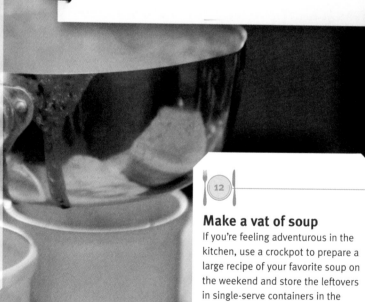

12

Make a vat of soup

If you're feeling adventurous in the kitchen, use a crockpot to prepare a large recipe of your favorite soup on the weekend and store the leftovers in single-serve containers in the freezer. Reheat the soup for lunch the next day or pair with a sandwich for a quick and easy weeknight meal.

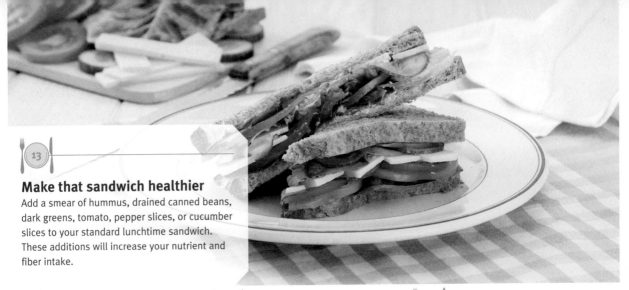

13

Make that sandwich healthier

Add a smear of hummus, drained canned beans, dark greens, tomato, pepper slices, or cucumber slices to your standard lunchtime sandwich. These additions will increase your nutrient and fiber intake.

14

Cooking in bulk

Bulk cooking and baking can prove to be a real time saver while also ensuring that you always have healthy meals on hand. Prepare larger servings of your favorite healthy foods and use them later in the week as leftovers or store in the freezer for a quick weeknight meal.

15

In a hurry?

Grab a can of low-sodium soup or a serving of homemade soup, and add 2 cups of mixed vegetables, spinach, or carrots to increase its nutritional value and help fill you up. Serve with a cheese sandwich on whole-wheat bread.

16

Minimize mess

There are some specific cooking methods that solo cooks can use to deliver fast and healthy meals at home without spending time on washing multiple dishes afterwards.

• **Sauté** a piece of meat in a skillet, add some vegetables, and pair with a whole grain such as brown rice for a quick and healthy one-pan meal.

• **Cooking in foil or parchment packets**, a method known as en papillote, uses steam to quickly and gently cook food without adding fat. Take a piece of fish or chicken, season it, add vegetables, and wrap it in foil or parchment. Simply place the packet in the oven and cook at the proper temperature. An added bonus to this method is that there are no pots and pans to clean up.

• **Roasting** is a simple cooking method that can save calories while delivering a healthy and delicious meal. Roast a small chicken or chicken breast, adding some vegetables such as carrots or turnips to the roasting pan.

Do this...

✓ Acknowledge that it's okay to prepare a meal for one, and that it can in fact be an enjoyable experience.

✓ Plan your meals. Scour the web and cooking magazines for low-calorie, delicious recipes. Variety ensures that you're getting more of the nutrients you need and keeps cooking interesting.

...Not this

✗ Fall into the trap of thinking that it's too much work to cook for one and eat convenience and take-out foods.

✗ Wait until hunger strikes to think about what you're going to eat. It's much more difficult to eat healthily if you're not prepared, and chances are you'll reach for the first thing you see!

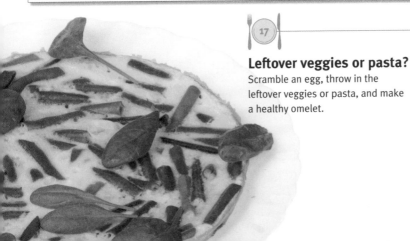

17

Leftover veggies or pasta?

Scramble an egg, throw in the leftover veggies or pasta, and make a healthy omelet.

18

Don't have time for a full dinner?

Enjoy breakfast at dinnertime. Breakfast foods are are good at any time, and are typically quick cooking and easy to prepare for just one person.

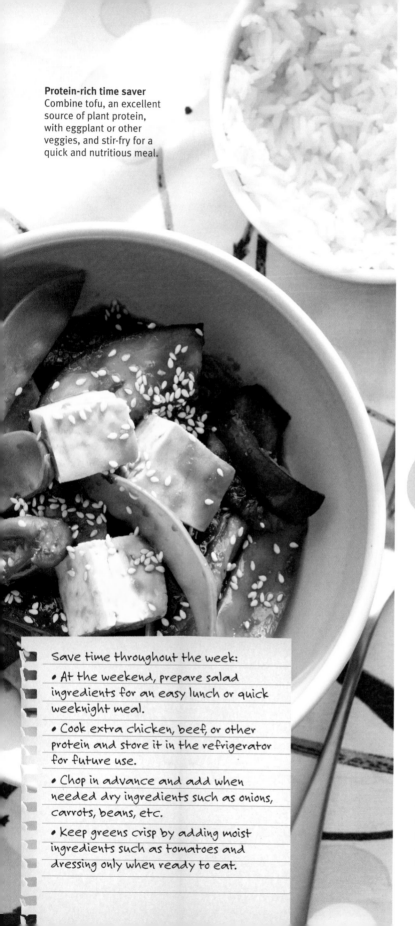

Protein-rich time saver
Combine tofu, an excellent source of plant protein, with eggplant or other veggies, and stir-fry for a quick and nutritious meal.

Save time throughout the week:
• At the weekend, prepare salad ingredients for an easy lunch or quick weeknight meal.
• Cook extra chicken, beef, or other protein and store it in the refrigerator for future use.
• Chop in advance and add when needed dry ingredients such as onions, carrots, beans, etc.
• Keep greens crisp by adding moist ingredients such as tomatoes and dressing only when ready to eat.

Enjoy the process

Enlist some mindful eating techniques, not only to save calories in home-prepared meals, but also to enhance the experience.

Before choosing your food check in and ask yourself what you really want to eat and consider how you want to feel after your meal.

Check ingredients labels: Are there fewer than 10 ingredients? Do you know what they all are and how they contribute to your nutrition intake, or otherwise?

Pause before and during your meal to assess your hunger level.

Pay attention to the colors, smells, tastes, and textures of your food.

Put your utensils down a few times during the meal to help you slow down.

> Before you sit down for a meal, do a short breathing exercise to become a more mindful eater. Breathe in for 4, hold for 7, and slowly exhale for 9 seconds. This foundation of being fully aware will help you overcome overeating.
>
> Cindy Guirino, Nutrition Writer and Consultant

 20

Have fun experimenting

When cooking for one, it's important to stay flexible and be prepared. Take note of which recipes work and which ones don't, as well as the flavors you like the most. Since you are cooking for yourself, you have more freedom to experiment. The good news is that you don't have to worry about anyone else liking your dish as you're the only one eating it!

Veggie pita pizza

We all like pizza. But store-bought pizza can be greasy and too big for one person. Enjoy the winning combination of cheese, dough, and tasty veggies with this perfectly sized version.

Ingredients
- 1 large whole-wheat pita bread
- 3–4 tbsp tomato sauce (to taste)
- 1 oz (30 g) shredded part-skim mozzarella cheese, chopped
- Assorted chopped vegetables

Directions
1. Preheat oven or toaster oven to 350°F (180°C).

2. Spread the tomato sauce on the pita and sprinkle with the cheese.

3. Add enough vegetables to cover the pita and bake for about 10 minutes or until the cheese is melted.

315 calories per serving (may vary based on vegetables used)

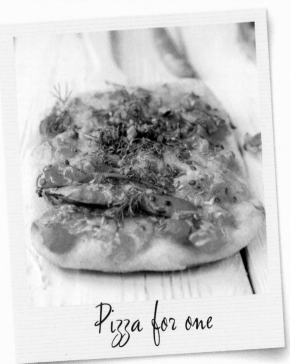

Pizza for one

A trip around the world in soup form

You can create an easy chicken and egg soup with different international flavors. Just boil 1–2 cups of chicken broth. Add one whisked egg and lightly heat until the egg is cooked (about one minute). Top with any of the following:

Mexican style Dash of hot pepper, chopped cilantro, and baked corn tortilla strips.

Greek style Teaspoon of lemon juice, a dash of olive oil, and chopped parsley.

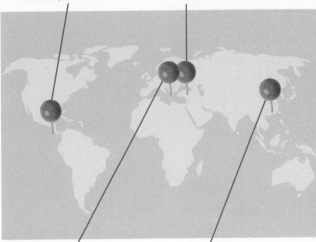

Italian style Chopped tomato, croûtons, oregano, and a dash of olive oil and garlic powder.

Chinese style Chopped scallions and 2 drops of sesame oil just before serving.

Check these out

www.allrecipes.com
Collection of recipes for solo cooks.
www.bbcgoodfood.com/recipes/collection/meals-one
Recipes for one, including cooking time and level of difficulty.

> Buy a whole boneless pork loin when it goes on sale. Have the butcher cut roasts, chops, and country ribs so you have a variety and save money.

Linda Eck Mills, Career and Life Coach

Cooking for many

Whether you have a large family or are planning a party, feeding many mouths—healthily—does not have to be a chore.

Cooking for many can be fun with some advance planning. All it takes is planning, preparation, and practice. Using those three "P"s will organize your work and guarantee your success in the kitchen—see below for more details.

If shopping to feed a family, stock up when key staples are on sale, buy in bulk where possible, and shop with the season to maximize freshness while minimizing cost.

Follow the three "P"s

Step 1: Planning

Think about the event itself and who will be coming. This will direct your efforts from the beginning. If it's a special event, what type of atmosphere do you want to create? Whether formal or informal, fun or serious, business or casual, all depends on your vision or goal for the event.

Think about what you will prepare, what you might ask friends or family members to prepare and bring, and what you can buy that doesn't require much preparation. At what time of day is the event or meal? Timing will greatly influence the type of foods you will serve. Do you need to serve a full meal or will hors d'œuvres suffice? You can save money by preparing some foods yourself but if time is at a premium, it may be worth buying some key elements pre-prepared (beware of "hidden" or dubious ingredients—see pages 64–67).

How much do you need per person?

Cooked vegetables	Beans	Green or leafy salads
½ cup per person if serving two vegetables (1–1½ cups for one vegetable or big eaters)	½ cup cooked beans per person (½–1 cup for vegetarians)	1–2 cups per person (2–3 cups per person if they like greens)

Store-cupboard staples
Be ready for a crowd and extend your meals with canned staples of low-sodium beans and veggies, water-packed tuna or chicken, and fruits packed in their own juice. Frozen options work well, too, if you have a good freezer.

Fruit, mixed	Grains	Cheese	Meat, poultry, or fish
½ cup per person (1 cup if it is a popular item)	½–1 cup or 1–2 oz (30–55 g) per person (3 oz [85 g] for heavy pasta or rice eaters or vegetarians who like grains)	1–2 oz (30–55 g) per person (more for lactovegetarians)	3 oz (85 g) per person (6 oz [170 g] for people who like meat, poultry, and fish; less than 3 oz [85 g] if you are serving more than one type of these items)

Step 2: Preparation

Before you start cooking, make a shopping/grocery list and check your pantry for staples you may already have on hand like dry pasta, brown or wild rice, barley or buckwheat groats, canned goods, drinks, or snack foods.

Organize your shopping list by the order of things you want to serve so you won't forget anything: appetizers, main dish, side dishes, salads, desserts, and beverages. Your time and money are valuable—don't waste them at the market. You want to enjoy your time at home cooking, not looking for ingredients.

Load your pantry with staples for quick and easy meals.
For example, with these items:
• low-sodium canned beans
• low-sodium canned vegetables
• tomato sauce or paste
• low-sodium chicken broth
• canned tuna, in water
• canned chicken, in water
• fruit packed in its own juice
...you can easily prepare any of the following:

1 Bean and veggie burgers

2 Chicken noodle soup

3 Fruit and nut dessert salad or snack

4 Minestrone soup

5 Barley and veggie salad

6 Pasta with marinara and vegetable sauce

7 Kasha with vegetables

8 Brown rice and beans

9 Wild rice with vegetables

10 Three-bean salad

Pull your recipes and think about what can be cooked or prepared in advance and where you will store it, and cooking times and methods to make sure you are aware of what you will need to do. Remember to thaw frozen foods a day in advance (in the refrigerator) to make sure they are ready for preparation.

Step 3: Practice

After you have had success with some of your large meals or events, you can recycle the recipes and cook them with confidence. Try variations of your recipes, in particular substituting lower-calorie ingredients or adding some healthy ones.

Examples of variations to try:
• Add flaxseeds, nuts, and dried fruit to salads
• Cut the fat by a third in recipes
• Use egg whites or egg substitutes
• Try baking usually "breaded and fried" favorites
• Add powdered dry milk to baked goods

 26

Be better equipped

Crockpots, stockpots, and electric skillets can give you more flexibility in the kitchen.

1 Leave dishes or sauces to simmer in crockpots or stockpots while you get on with something else.

2 Use an electric skillet for convenient sautéing, grilling, or for omelets and frittatas.

3 Switch to the low heat function to keep food warm when hosting an event.

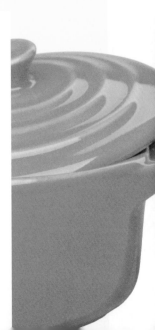

27

Useful hints and tips when cooking for many

Save time and calories with appetizers and snacks by serving a variety of nuts, raw fruits and vegetables, and salads to balance higher-calorie foods to come later in the menu.

Cook sweet potatoes in the microwave. Cool, cut into sticks, toss lightly with cinnamon and brown sugar (just a light scattering), and "oven-fry."

Make a large batch of macaroni or other similar-shaped pasta. Lightly sauté fresh chopped kale and mushrooms in olive oil and garlic. Mix and serve.

Stretch the meat dollars and make dishes healthier by cooking fricassées and stews with a tomato sauce or low-sodium broth base with mostly celery, carrots, onions, tomatoes, and potatoes (with skin) and less meat or chicken.

Set up a pizza, taco, or other fun "bar" where your guests can serve themselves. Warm up whole-wheat pitas or whole-grain taco shells and set out healthy toppings such as beans, vegetables, low-fat cheese, and even fruit.

28

Three dishes to cook for picky eaters

Pick a base dish and include two or three side items your choosy eaters can select from:

1 Taco base: Prepare seasoned lean ground beef served with a choice of soft corn and whole-wheat tortillas, leafy greens, chopped tomatoes and peppers, grated low-fat cheese, and taco sauce.

2 Pasta base: Prepare whole-wheat pasta served with a choice of chickpeas, grilled tuna, chicken chunks, cherry tomatoes, chopped fresh herbs, and 2–3 low-fat dressings.

3 Brown rice, barley, or quinoa base: Prepare the rice or quinoa served with a choice of black beans, corn, chopped onions and peppers, olives, chopped parsley or basil, lemon, and olive oil.

Do this...

✓ Broil or bake meats for more efficient use of your preparation time and to reduce fat and calories.

...Not this

✗ Fry meats. This requires more of your "watch time" (you have to stand over it constantly) and adds fat and calories.

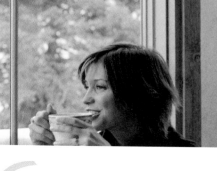

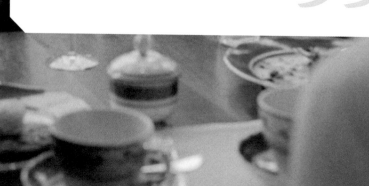

" Cooking for many? Prepare dishes that are made in advance, can be kept hot or cold during the event— with minimal work from you—and require self-service. This frees you up to enjoy the company. "

Dr. Judith Rodriguez, Professor and Registered Dietitian, University of North Florida

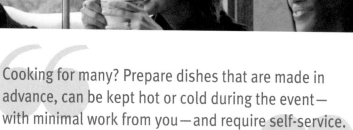

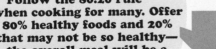

80%

Follow the 80:20 rule when cooking for many. Offer 80% healthy foods and 20% that may not be so healthy—the overall meal will be a satisfying mix of nutrients and treats.

20%

 30

Three ideas for healthier dishes to make in advance

1 **Make a big batch of chili** by using more beans than meat and a combination of tofu crumbles and lean ground beef or turkey.

2 **Make a big batch of tortellini or gnocchi**, and season with olive oil and fresh herbs. A few hours before serving, toss in washed and chopped broccoli and cauliflower (or a few bags of frozen). Reheat, toss, and top with grated cheese before serving.

3 **Make your own meatballs** by mixing half-ground beef and half-moistened whole-wheat bread (use broth or water to moisten) with egg whites and seasonings.

 29

Check these out

www.dummies.com/how-to/content/cooking-for-crowds-for-dummies-cheat-sheet.html
Includes a chart to help you find out how much food you need to prepare.

www.pinterest.com/juzt4j/recipes-to-feed-a-crowd
Recipe ideas for crowds, ranging from appetizers to desserts.

31   serves **5**

Salad for all seasons

A quick, easy, and healthy salad can be made with mixed greens, chopped or dried fruit, nuts, and cheese.

Ingredients

- 5 cups mixed greens
- ¼ cup chopped dried cranberries, cherries, or apricots
- ¼ cup chopped or sliced walnuts, peanuts, or almonds
- ¼ cup crumbled Gorgonzola cheese

Directions

Put the greens in the bottom of the salad bowl. Sprinkle with the dried fruit, nuts, and crumbled cheese. Add the salad dressing (see right) before serving, or serve on the side of the salad.

All-seasons salad dressing

Use one quarter of this dressing for your salad; save the rest for later!

Ingredients

- ½ cup orange juice
- 3 tbsp olive oil
- 1 tbsp balsamic vinegar
- ½ tsp pepper
- ½ tsp dill weed
- 2 packets Splenda (or other sugar substitute)

Directions

Place the ingredients in a shaker bottle or whisk together in a bowl and serve over the salad.

126 calories per serving of salad with dressing

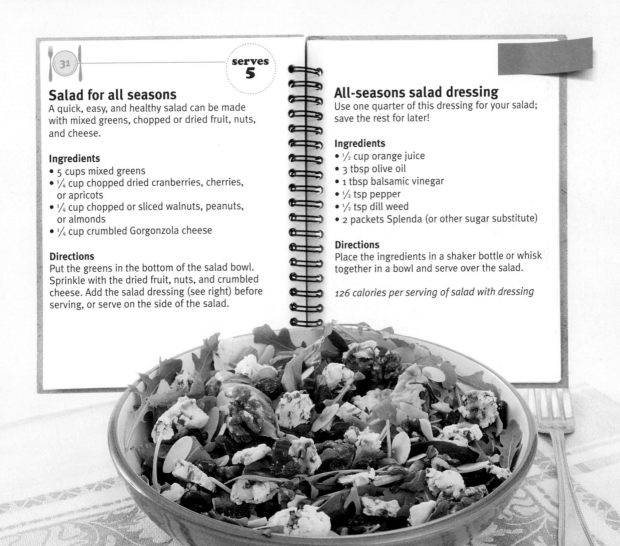

Breakfast: Kick-start your health goals

Breakfast is your first opportunity of the day to work toward your weight and health goals.

1 Brain: Needs energy in the form of glucose, primarily provided by carbohydrates.

2 Heart: Protein, calcium, sodium, potassium, and other nutrients are important for a healthy heart.

3 Lungs: Vitamins C and E are antioxidants that support lung health.

4 Stomach: An important muscle that needs protein and vitamins.

5 Kidneys: Water and adequate—but not excessive—amounts of minerals are important for renal health.

6 Intestines: Need fiber and adequate fluids for gut health.

By definition, breakfast can be at any time of the day, if it is a time when you "break a fast," that is, start to eat after an extended period of not eating. But traditionally it is used to refer to the first meal after awakening from a long, hopefully restful, sleep. The key point about breakfast is to eat something that will provide energy to "get you going" and also key nutrients and satiety (fullness) value. Feeling full will help you manage your appetite throughout the day. Breakfast is important for children to help them learn while at school, and important for adults to help them concentrate on the task at hand, whatever that might be.

Treat your body

A good breakfast contains a combination of carbohydrates in the form of starches for energy and fiber for gut health, and protein to build and support your tissues and organs throughout the day. A small amount of the healthy fats will help with the feeling of fullness. But you also want to

TOP 10 HEALTHY power breakfasts

1
Whole-grain or high-fiber dry cereal with low-fat or fat-free milk; fruit or glass of juice.

2
Hard-boiled egg; English muffin with a slice of cheese; cup of tea.

3
Piece of leftover chicken breast on whole-wheat toast; glass of juice.

4
Cold noodles with peanut sauce and tofu; glass of water.

5
Pita bread with hummus; side salad of chopped tomatoes; olives; glass of water.

6
Oatmeal made with low-fat milk, topped with peaches; cup of coffee.

7
Shredded wheat cereal with low fat milk; apple; cup of herbal tea.

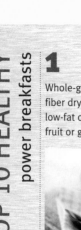
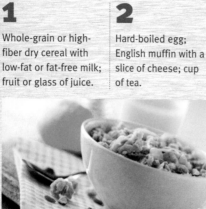
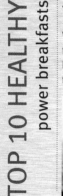

include nutrients that will allow your body to function well throughout the day. The micronutrients—vitamins and minerals—and phytochemicals—natural chemicals found in plant foods—help to regulate important body functions and promote health.

 32

Meal replacers

There are commercial beverages or food bars available called "meal replacers." For people who are trying to lose weight, meal replacers provide two important components dieters want: a known number of calories and some key nutrients.

 33

Plan ahead

Select two breakfast items and place them prominently in the kitchen. Position the whole-wheat bread next to the coffee pot, and the yogurt at the front of the eye-level refrigerator shelf. That way, you won't be tempted by other foods en route.

 34

How many calories should I eat for breakfast?

While currently there is no set rule, the key is to determine your eating pattern and then allot a portion of those calories for breakfast.

- ■ Breakfast
- ■ Lunch
- ■ Dinner
- ■ Snack or light meal

Eat only three meals and not snack throughout the day? If so, break your calories up into thirds. For example, if your goal is to eat 1,800 calories a day, you may want to make your breakfast 500–600 calories.

Eat three meals and two snacks a day? If so, consider breaking your calories up into three large and two smaller calorie distributions. For example, if your goal is to eat 1,800 calories a day, you may want to make your meals 400–500 calories and each of your two snacks 100–150 calories a day.

Eat about six small meals or large snacks; that is, graze for most of the day? Then you might want to have about 300 calories per meal/snack.

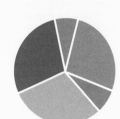

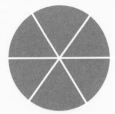

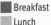

COUNTDOWN COUNTER

EGG BREAKFAST | CALORIES

1 hard-cooked egg, 1 glass orange juice, plain whole-wheat toast | **272 calories**

1 fried egg, 1 glass orange juice, whole-wheat toast with butter | **318 calories**

1 egg Benedict, 1 glass orange juice, whole-wheat toast with butter and jam | **637 calories**

GENERAL BREAKFAST OPTIONS | CALORIES

8 oz plain Greek yogurt topped with 1 cup canned drained peaches, ¼ cup granola, herbal tea | **342 calories**

1 cup bran cereal with raisins, 1% milk, fresh orange, plain tea | **355 calories**

6-inch whole-wheat pancake topped with ½ cup unsweetened applesauce, 1 slice grilled Canadian-style bacon, plain coffee | **445 calories**

1 cup low-fat granola (no raisins), 1 glass skim/nonfat milk, 1 cup strawberries, 1 glass orange juice | **450 calories**

8

Bagel topped with a slice of smoked salmon and onion; cup of coffee.

9

Cinnamon scone; cube of Cheddar cheese; wedge of honeydew melon; cup of tea.

10

Fruit and yogurt smoothie; granola bar; glass of water.

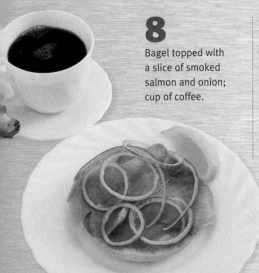

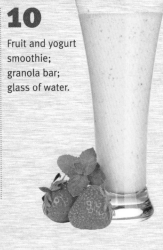

Make time for lunch

Whether you are in a hurry or taking your time, at home or at work, lunch is an important meal that can refuel you.

Lunch is the meal that gets you over that midday "hump" to provide you with energy until later in the day.

Meals tend to be larger for people with physically demanding jobs such as farm work, and smaller meals are generally consumed by people with sedentary jobs such as office work, but it depends on your eating habits and, in particular, the size and times of your other meals and snacks (see page 27).

Lunch also varies around the world. In some areas, it is a multi-course meal consumed slowly, as a major social event or the main meal of the day. In other areas, it may be light, consisting of bread or other starch and a high-protein food. Brunch has also become popular, describing a late breakfast or early lunch that has the elements of both meals. It is most common on weekends.

What's your goal?
Consider how you want to feel after you eat. Rested? Energized? Avoid skipping the meal, since it will make you feel tired, moody, or irritable (it's hard to be nice when you are hungry and have low blood sugar). A combination of complex carbohydrates and proteins will rejuvenate the mind and body. Stimulants such as coffee may perk you up temporarily, especially if combined with sugar, but this is followed by a blood sugar drop, and too much caffeine could make you nervous and irritable.

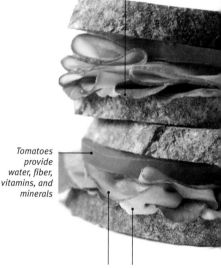

Whole-wheat bread for fiber, to keep you feeling fuller for longer

Add leafy greens at every opportunity, for vitamins and minerals

Tomatoes provide water, fiber, vitamins, and minerals

Sliced turkey for lean protein, to replenish and rebuild

Add a bit of cheese for protein (curbs hunger) and calcium (for bone health)

 35

Brown-bag lunch

While some people will eat lunch at restaurants or eateries near their place of work, this pattern is facing competition from the traditional "brown bag" lunch, when people prepare lunch at home and bring it to work. If you work at a location that has a cafeteria, the food lines may be long, or the food not to your liking—or preferred quality or price range. This may be the same with food from local restaurants, and sitting down in a restaurant may be too time consuming in the first place. When you brown-bag your lunch, you undoubtedly save money, but you also have more control over flavor and your time, and can feel comforted that you know the quality of the ingredients.

 36

Three brown-bag time-saving tips

1 Make five sandwiches at a time, and freeze each in individual freezer bags.

2 Cook a large dinner and set some aside in a lunch container.

3 Include individually wrapped cheese, crackers, and fruit cups in small plastic bags.

What does lunch mean to you?

Something quick to eat while running errands or working? Watch out for hidden calories in quick-serve pre-prepared foods.

Something low-cost? Try "brown bagging" meals (see opposite).

The best choice at a quick-service eatery? Focus on the smart choices regarding portion size and side items.

The best choice at your work cafeteria? Try the simple items, like grilled chicken and salad instead of mixed dishes such as casseroles.

Something you eat out while sharing time with friends or colleagues? Consider splitting the meal—and cost—or having an appetizer instead of a full meal.

38

Focus your mind

Interestingly enough, although people may feel that it is a fast meal, lunch actually tends to be one of the longer meals. This may be because people are often distracted talking to friends or working while eating lunch. They may feel like it did not take much time to eat or have a feeling of satisfaction. This mindless eating pattern can lead to overeating. Stop, take time to eat (instead of multitasking), and enjoy the meal and break from work or the day's routine.

> When you sit down to eat, take a couple of deep breaths, relax, look at your food, and tell yourself, 'I'm going to relax, eat, and enjoy my food.' This can help you slow down, focus on the experience of eating, and eat less.

Penny L. Wilson, www.eatingforperformance.com

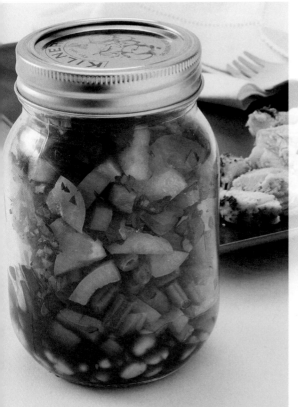

39

Lunch in a jar

Get a 16 oz (450 g) or larger Mason jar and add:

- 2 tablespoons of your favorite salad dressing
- Any "hard" veggies: coarsely chopped carrots, broccoli, cooked beets, etc., or cooked beans
- Any "medium" veggies: chopped green beans or snap peas, green, yellow, or red peppers, etc.
- Any "light" veggies: chopped greens, cabbage, etc.
- Protein such as chicken pieces (leftovers) or cheese

Directions

Pour the dressing into the Mason jar. Add the hard chopped veggies, followed by the medium, then light veggies. Seal the jar. Just before serving, shake the jar to mix the ingredients. Arrange on a plate and top with the protein.

COUNTDOWN COUNTER

?

LUNCH ITEM | CALORIES

Steamed broccoli, 1 cup | **27 calories**

Turkey breast, 1 oz (28 g) | **34 calories**

Honeydew melon, 1 cup | **64 calories**

Beef salami, 1 oz | **74 calories**

Medium banana | **105 calories**

Hummus, ¼ cup | **109 calories**

Cheddar cheese, 1 oz (28 g) | **113 calories**

Medium potato, baked or microwaved | **145 calories**

White bread, 2 slices | **160 calories**

1 pita bread | **170 calories**

Peanut butter, 2 tbsp | **190 calories**

Berry-flavored yogurt, 1 cup | **233 calories**

Medium oat bran bagel | **268 calories**

Dinner: The healthy option

Dinner is the opportunity to enjoy the last meal of the day, and make sure you've had your daily dose of nutrients.

Dinner is usually the last meal of the day, eaten around 6pm or later in the evening in many countries. For most people, dinner is based on convenience but is still more elaborate than breakfast and lunch. Dinner is a great opportunity to get creative with ingredients and flavors but, in reality, people often have limited time to prepare dinner and can feel hungry and tired after a hard day at work, and so may not always make healthy choices.

Build a well-balanced dinner

You should aim to include each food group in your dinner. As with breakfast (see pages 26–27) and lunch (see pages 28–29), a complete meal should consist of carbohydrates, protein, and a small amount of healthy fats. All of these macronutrients are needed for energy (carbohydrates, fat) and healthy tissue growth and maintenance (protein, fat). It is recommended that these three key macronutrients are obtained from high-

fiber starches, grains, fruits, and vegetables (carbohydrates); lean meats, fish, poultry, or plant proteins (protein); and heart-healthy oils such as extra virgin olive oil and canola oil (fat). An example of a well-balanced dinner meal is the following:
• ²/₃ cup wild rice
• 3 oz (85 g) baked wild salmon
• 1 cup steamed green beans

Check your food groups

Your dinner portions should be adjusted according to how much of each food group you have already eaten throughout the day. Therefore, dinner is a great occasion for including food groups that you may have missed throughout the day, or an opportunity to cut down on food groups of which you may have already met your limits. For example:
• If you did not have any **vegetables or fruit** for breakfast and/or lunch, catch up at dinnertime. Since fruits and vegetables provide important nutrients such as vitamins, minerals, antioxidants, and fiber, which all help ward off diseases, they are recommended to be eaten every day.
• Likewise, if you had a large lunch, which included a foot-long meatball sandwich, it would be best to go easy on the amount of **protein** for dinner. Instead of 3 oz (85 g) of salmon, have only 1 oz (30 g) for dinner, with increased vegetables.

Dinner plate composition

There are several ways of deciding on portion sizes. One easy approach is the New American Plate from the American Institute for Cancer Research. This approach suggests that two thirds (or more) of your plate should be made up of vegetables, fruits, whole grains, or beans, and one third (or less) of animal protein. Another similar approach from the United States Department of Agriculture named My Plate is shown to the right. These methods are mere guidelines and you must keep in mind that you may need to adjust your dinner portions depending on what you already ate throughout the day.

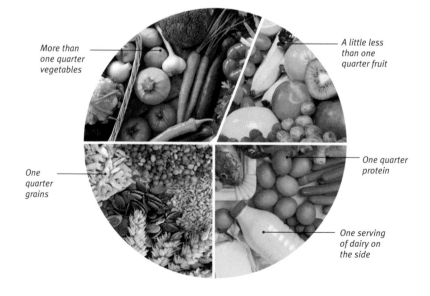

More than one quarter vegetables

A little less than one quarter fruit

One quarter grains

One quarter protein

One serving of dairy on the side

Building blocks of a healthy, complete dinner

Grains and starches for carbohydrates

| Brown or wild rice | Whole-wheat or whole-grain pasta | Bread, tortillas | Whole-grain quinoa | Red potatoes, with skin | Sweet potatoes |

The longer the shelf life, the shorter your life. Eat real food!

Vegetables that are high in carbohydrates

While these vegetables do contain a great amount of nutrition, they also contain as much starch as grains. They should be considered a carbohydrate and not a regular vegetable.

| Potatoes | Sweet potatoes | Peas | Corn | Pumpkin | Butternut and acorn squash | Yams |

Vegetables low in carbohydrates and calories

All of these are good choices. Try to eat as many different vegetables throughout the week as possible. If there are some you have not tried before, give them a try—you might be pleasantly surprised!

| Broccoli | Green beans | Cauliflower | Cabbage | Eggplant | Carrots | Salad greens | Tomatoes |

 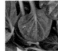   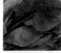 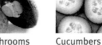

| Kohlrabi | Spinach | Bell peppers | Onions | Leeks | Garlic | Mushrooms | Cucumbers |

| Zucchini | Summer squash | Radishes | Brussels sprouts |

Good protein choices

Lean beef, pork, lamb, etc. with all visible fat trimmed off and no marbling. Lean poultry includes chicken and turkey breast, without the skin. Other parts of poultry have a higher fat content. Fish—in particular, fatty fish such as salmon and trout—is a healthy choice since it contains great amounts of omega-3 fatty acids, which are beneficial for numerous body functions, including protection of heart health.

     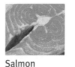

| Beef | Pork | Lamb | Chicken | Turkey | Salmon | Trout |

Oil-less preparation methods

While fried foods may taste good, they add unnecessary calories and fat. There are many healthy alternative methods to frying such as:
• Baking
• Broiling
• Grilling
• Lightly sautéing
• Steaming
Some of these methods require the use of little or no oil. If some oil is needed, aim for canola or sunflower oil. But use sparingly, as oils contain about 120 calories per tablespoon. You can also use extra virgin olive oil to drizzle over salads or steamed vegetables. According to the American Heart Association, you should avoid coconut oil, palm oil, and palm kernel oil. While these are vegetable oils and have no cholesterol, they are high in saturated fat.

Eat dinner early

Aim to eat dinner earlier in the evening rather than later whenever you can. Researchers suggest that this will give your body the opportunity to properly digest your food. Unwanted pounds are also less likely to creep up so this strategy may help with weight loss if that is your goal. Furthermore, by eating dinner earlier in the evening you also avoid heartburn, which can be triggered by lying down shortly after eating. According to the National Institute of Health, it is recommended to avoid lying down for at least three to four hours after eating.

Green is good
A starter salad should comprise mostly greens. Consider adding low-calorie and filling veggies such as broccoli, celery, or green beans. Sprinkle with a flavored vinegar.

A light start

Studies have shown that eating a low-calorie soup or salad before the main course results in a significant reduction of energy intake during the remainder of the meal. However, these soups and salads must be light in calories, otherwise you could easily overdo it. Good examples of first-course salads are leafy-green, colorful salads consisting of only vegetables (no protein such as chicken or beans—those salads should be considered a main course). Filling yet energy-light soups are broth or chunky vegetable soup. This is not only an easy way to increase your vegetable and fiber intake, but this will also help to avoid overeating with the rest of your dinner, because you will feel satisfied more quickly.

TOP 10 TIPS for dinnertime success

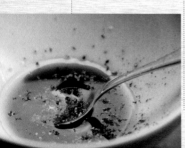

1
Make a menu for the week or for several days. Then shop for the required items in one or two trips to avoid having to go out every day.

2
Plan and prepare ahead. Wash and chop ingredients that can withstand being prepped ahead of time (bell peppers, broccoli, green beans, cabbage, etc.) so they are ready to use when needed.

3
Marinate the night before if the recipe calls for it, and also to infuse flavor.

4
Buy certain items in bulk that you can pre-prep and freeze. For example, sauté a quantity of lean ground beef, use half for one dinner, and freeze the rest for another night. Or buy a large quantity of chicken breast, trim (if needed), portion out, and freeze.

5
Use produce that is in season. It is not only packed with more flavor and nutrients, but is also usually cheaper.

6
Keep your kitchen pantry stocked with staples such as brown rice, whole-wheat pasta, canned beans, tomato sauce, low-sodium soup, fruit cups in 100% juice, etc.

7
Keep some frozen or canned fruits and vegetables on hand for convenience. Use no-salt-added or low-sodium for canned vegetables. Rinse before using. Canned fruits should be packed in water or 100% juice with no sugar added.

47

A quick way to cook potatoes

Microwave potatoes instead of boiling or baking them. Wash and pierce the potatoes. Microwave them for about three to six minutes (depending on their size and quantity) until they are slightly soft. Then wrap them in foil and let them sit to steam and continue cooking. You can have perfectly cooked potatoes in less time than baking and with more nutrient retention than boiling.

48

Check these out

www.eatingwell.com/recipes_menus
A treasure trove of healthy recipes, incuding one-pot recipes for easy weeknight meals.

www.realsimple.com/food-recipes
Plenty of ideas for easy weeknight dinners.

www.cookinglight.com/food/quick-healthy
Healthy and fast recipes for busy people.

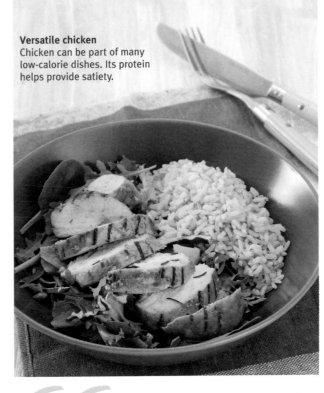

Versatile chicken
Chicken can be part of many low-calorie dishes. Its protein helps provide satiety.

> "The weekend (Friday dinner–Sunday dinner) has over 30% of your meals for the week. Do you want to eat healthily only 67% of the time?"

Kathleen Searles, Nutrition Consultant, www.lunchbox-nutritionist.com

8

Seek out one-pot meals—you will have less to clean up afterward when your entire dinner can be prepared in just one pot or pan. Casseroles and slow-cooker recipes can save you lots of time. So try different one-pot recipes such as green bean casserole with chicken baked in condensed low-sodium mushroom soup, pinto bean and chicken sausage stew, tuna noodle casserole, and macaroni cheese with a layer of spinach. Many of these kinds of recipes can be found online.

9

Stop by the grocery store on your way home from work and pick up a rotisserie chicken, bag of pre-washed salad greens, a few tomatoes, 1 small cucumber, baby carrots, and a small whole-grain baguette. At home, quickly chop the vegetables and toss with the salad greens with a drizzle of olive oil and vinegar or your favorite dressing with the shredded chicken breast on top. Toast the baguette and lightly dip in extra virgin olive oil sprinkled with dried basil and oregano (or any other herbs or spices you love).

10

Combining snacks to make a meal—when your fridge is almost empty and you are too tired to go to the grocery store, let alone cook—doesn't mean you have to skimp on nutrition. Have some whole-grain cereal or oats with skim or low-fat milk combined with a handful of baby carrots and some fruit, and you have a wholesome meal. Or have your favorite low-sodium soup with some toasted whole-grain bread. Keep a few fruit cups packed in 100% juice in your store-cupboard for when you are running low on time and energy.

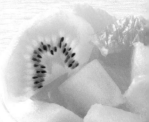

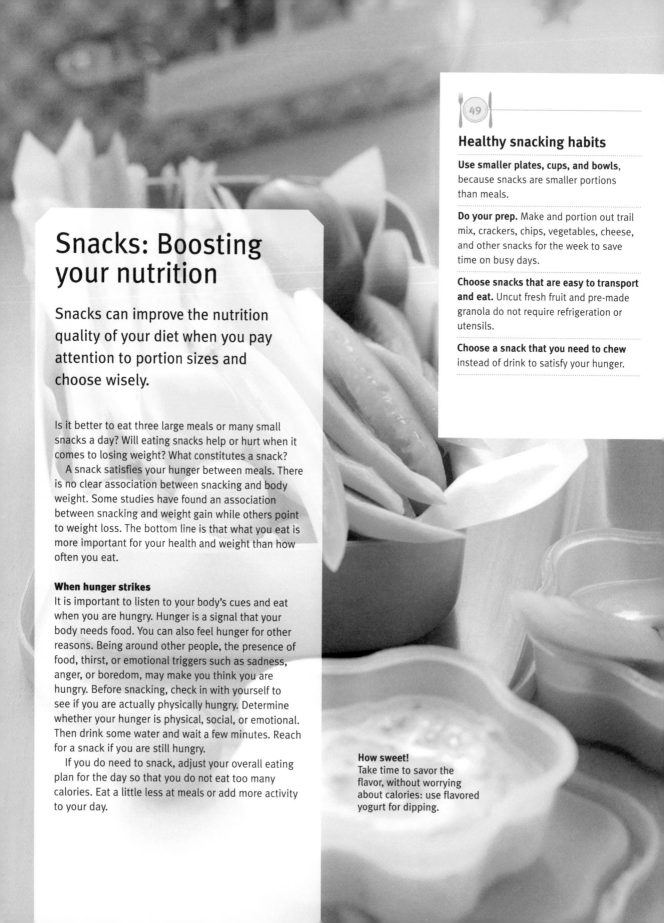

Snacks: Boosting your nutrition

Snacks can improve the nutrition quality of your diet when you pay attention to portion sizes and choose wisely.

Is it better to eat three large meals or many small snacks a day? Will eating snacks help or hurt when it comes to losing weight? What constitutes a snack?

A snack satisfies your hunger between meals. There is no clear association between snacking and body weight. Some studies have found an association between snacking and weight gain while others point to weight loss. The bottom line is that what you eat is more important for your health and weight than how often you eat.

When hunger strikes

It is important to listen to your body's cues and eat when you are hungry. Hunger is a signal that your body needs food. You can also feel hunger for other reasons. Being around other people, the presence of food, thirst, or emotional triggers such as sadness, anger, or boredom, may make you think you are hungry. Before snacking, check in with yourself to see if you are actually physically hungry. Determine whether your hunger is physical, social, or emotional. Then drink some water and wait a few minutes. Reach for a snack if you are still hungry.

If you do need to snack, adjust your overall eating plan for the day so that you do not eat too many calories. Eat a little less at meals or add more activity to your day.

Healthy snacking habits

Use smaller plates, cups, and bowls, because snacks are smaller portions than meals.

Do your prep. Make and portion out trail mix, crackers, chips, vegetables, cheese, and other snacks for the week to save time on busy days.

Choose snacks that are easy to transport and eat. Uncut fresh fruit and pre-made granola do not require refrigeration or utensils.

Choose a snack that you need to chew instead of drink to satisfy your hunger.

How sweet!
Take time to savor the flavor, without worrying about calories: use flavored yogurt for dipping.

Filling the gaps

Use snacks to round out your nutrition. A snack that will satisfy your hunger for longer contains protein, fat, and/or fiber. Including at least two of these nutrients in each snack will give you more staying power.

QUICK GUIDE
to nutrients
Protein
Meats, dairy products, nuts, beans, seeds
....
Fats
Oils and spreads, nuts and seeds, avocado
....
Fiber
Whole grains, beans, fruit, vegetables
....

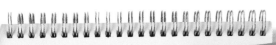

> Blend equal amounts of non-fat Greek yogurt with the following to cut calories and fat in half: guacamole, hummus, ranch dressing, blue cheese dressing, mayo in tuna salad or chicken salad or potato salad.

Georgia Kostas, Author, *The Cooper Clinic Solution to the Diet Revolution: Step Up to the Plate!*

Roasted chickpeas

This recipe is budget-friendly, packed with protein and fiber, and provides an easily portable snack.

Ingredients
- Chickpeas, boiled (or canned, rinsed)
- Your choice of spices (e.g., paprika, cayenne pepper, cumin, garlic powder, salt)
- Non-stick cooking spray

Directions
1. Preheat the oven to 450°F (230°C). Prepare the dried chickpeas as directed and drain, or rinse canned chickpeas.

2. Place wet chickpeas and spices in a plastic bag, seal, and shake to cover the chickpeas with the spices.

3. Spray a cookie sheet with non-stick cooking spray and spread the chickpeas in a single layer on the baking sheet. Place in a preheated oven and cook until crunchy, approximately 30–45 minutes, shaking the baking sheet occasionally to prevent sticking.

Serving suggestion: Enjoy a ½ cup serving on its own or add to homemade trail mix or on top of a salad for a protein-rich crunch.

176 calories, 7 g protein, 6 g fiber per ½ cup serving

Tempting treats

Be aware that prepackaged snack foods may be high in calories and low in nutrition. These are typically high in fat and sodium, or salt, and low in vitamins, minerals, and fiber. As a smart snacker, do allow yourself to enjoy a snack just for fun—chocolate, chips, or cake—but only have these as occasional treats and keep portions small.

Did you know celery sticks stay crisp for longer after you cut them if you store them in a cup of water in the fridge?

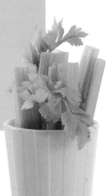

COUNTDOWN COUNTER

SNACK | CALORIES

Air-popped popcorn, 4 cups | **80 calories**

Reduced-fat Greek yogurt with peach, 5 oz (140 g) | **125 calories**

Roasted chickpeas, ½ cup | **135 calories**

12 baked tortilla chips with 2 tablespoons salsa | **140 calories**

Whole-grain cereal, 1 cup, with handful of raisins | **150 calories**

Dark chocolate, 1 oz (30 g) | **155 calories**

Almonds, 1 oz (30 g) | **160 calories**

14 pita chips with 2 tablespoons hummus | **195 calories**

Reduced-fat Swiss cheese, 2 oz (55 g), on 6 whole-grain crackers | **200 calories**

2 tablespoons peanut butter on 2 large celery stalks | **230 calories**

Bag of pretzels, 2 oz (55 g) | **280 calories**

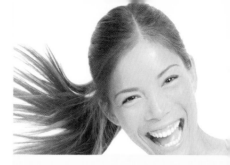

Getting and staying active

Even if you don't have access to a gym or equipment, there are many ways you can still get all the benefits of exercise while at home.

You know it's something you should do. And you probably know why: Moving and being active are critical for maintaining good health. Inactivity is as much of a health risk as any of the other major risk factors—such as smoking—for the development of chronic diseases.

The decision to become more active is life changing. Your quality of life will increase; quite possibly the risk of developing heart disease, diabetes, and stroke will diminish; as could the risk of developing high blood pressure and high cholesterol. Physical activity plays an important role in any weight-loss program; when you exercise, your body uses more calories than you eat and you lose weight. Also, your mood

will improve. You will sleep better, have more energy, feel less stress and anxiety, tone your muscles, and decrease the risk of osteoporosis. Why wouldn't you want all these rewards and positive feelings in your life?

There are three areas of fitness that you need to focus on:
• Flexibility
• Cardiovascular or aerobic fitness
• Muscular strength and endurance

These three areas of fitness do not require costly gym memberships or even leaving the house. You can do many if not most activities in the comfort of your own home. Some you can even do at work!

> " Start small and make it enjoyable. Try to do some fun physical activity every day by making it part of your daily routine. If it's fun, your activity choices will soon become your healthy lifestyle habits.

Chris Robertson, Assistant Professor of Exercise Science, Jacksonville University

53

Consult your doctor

Before you start any kind of exercise regimen, make sure that you consult a doctor for medical clearance. This is especially important if you are a male over 45 years of age or a female over 55 years of age. There is no condition that exercise can worsen, as long as it is the right kind of exercise done in a safe way.

54

Set realistic goals

Once you have been given the all-clear from your doctor, set one or two short-term and long-term realistic goals for yourself.
• **As a short-term goal: Less sitting!** While watching your favorite TV show, walk in place or do some stretching exercises.
• **As a long-term goal: Decrease leisure time spent at the computer** by at least half. You will find yourself with more time for exercising and should also feel less lethargic.

55

Make exercise a lifestyle routine

Make an "appointment" to exercise. Schedule exercise as you would any other important activity. This will integrate it into your life, making it a lifelong habit.

Get past those relapses: Everyone has relapses. But there's a difference between a relapse and giving up. Not exercising for a month after you've been exercising for three months may be a relapse. It doesn't mean you're a failure and you should not give up. Do not feel guilty—think of it as a time to reflect. Ask yourself, what happened? Why did you stop exercising? Think of ways to get yourself going again. Learn from your relapse so that you can keep on moving toward your goal of staying physically active. It is important to keep at it, even if you slip up or have relapses along the way.

Congratulate yourself! Remember to congratulate yourself for fitting activity into your day. After you finish your exercise, take a few minutes to reflect on how good it made you feel and use this to motivate yourself to continue exercising. When you achieve a long-term goal, give yourself an external reward too, such as treating yourself to a movie, a new outfit, new walking shoes, a pedometer, or tickets to a special event.

Exercise effectiveness: Calorie burning

The chart below gives calorie-burning estimates for popular sports and household chores. As you become more fit and do the activity more efficiently you will expend fewer calories. However, as you become more fit you will be able to exercise for longer and more vigorously.

BODY WEIGHT LB/KG	100/45	120/54	140/64	160/73	180/82	200/91	210/95
EXERCISE	calories burned per hour	calories burned per hour	calories burned per hour	calories burned per hour	calories burned per hour	calories burned per hour	calories burned per hour
Aerobics, high impact	332	398	465	531	598	664	697
Aerobics, low impact	228	274	319	365	410	456	479
Aerobics, in water	251	301	351	402	452	502	527
Walking, 2 mph (3 kmph)	128	154	179	205	230	256	269
Walking, 3.5 mph (5.5 kmph)	196	235	274	314	353	392	412
Running, 5 mph (8 kmph)	378	454	529	605	680	756	794
Cycling, 10 mph (16 kmph)	182	218	255	291	328	364	382
Tennis, singles	264	317	370	422	475	528	554
Weightlifting, general	156	187	218	250	281	312	328
Swimming, laps	264	317	370	422	475	528	554
Yoga, dynamic	396	475	554	634	713	792	832
Rowing, stationary	273	328	382	437	491	546	573
DOMESTIC CHORE/ACTIVITY							
Cooking	120	144	168	192	216	240	252
Dusting	134	161	188	214	241	268	281
Cleaning	159	191	223	254	286	318	334
Mopping floors	204	245	286	326	367	408	428
Gardening	182	218	255	291	328	364	382
Dancing, energetic	252	302	353	403	454	504	529
Vacuuming	167	200	233	267	300	333	350
Washing car	204	245	286	326	367	408	428
Washing dishes	102	122	143	163	184	204	214

Stretches for flexibility

Flexibility is the ability to move your joints and muscles within their entire range of motion. Performing stretching exercises will increase blood flow throughout the body, help burn calories, and decrease overall pain while increasing overall flexibility. And, even better news, stretches can be done easily in the home with little or no equipment.

Lower back and hip stretch: Lie on your back. Bring both knees to your chest and roll to the left and right. Bring both legs back to the center and release them down to the floor. Then pull one knee at a time up to the chest, holding each leg there for about 3 seconds.

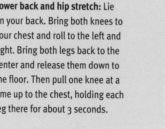

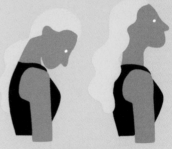

Neck stretch: Slowly lower your chin to your chest. Bring it back to a resting position. Next, move your head to the right and tilt your ear toward that shoulder. Make sure you keep both shoulders down. You will feel the stretch along the left side of your neck. Bring your head back to its resting position then repeat the same motion to the left by tilting your left ear to your left shoulder. Slowly repeat this exercise several times.

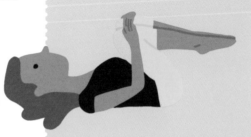

Aerobic activities to do at home

When you are aerobically fit, your cardiovascular and respiratory system effectively move oxygen around the body. When you are doing aerobic exercise your heart is beating faster and you are breathing harder. For these exercises, wear low-heeled shoes with traction, such as gym shoes. Continue exercising until you feel slightly out of breath, gradually increasing the amount of time that is spent on the activity.

Stepping: This exercise is ideal on stairs or steps. Lift one foot and place it on the lowest step, then lift the second foot to join the first foot on the step. Make sure you are well balanced or holding onto a stair rail or wall. Return the first foot back to the ground, followed by the second foot. Repeat, gradually increasing your pace.

Marching in place: Before you begin, you should feel balanced. Use support if needed; a counter top or the back of a chair. Raise one leg, making sure that your knee is level with your hip, or as high as you can but not beyond hip level or where you feel discomfort. Return that leg to the floor and repeat with the other leg. Do this as fast as you can without compromising your balance.

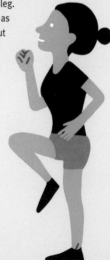

59

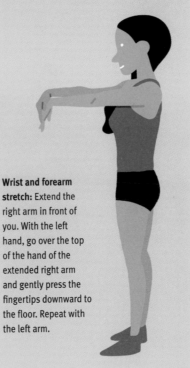

Arm across the chest stretch: Straighten one arm in front of you, grasp it just above the tricep (the muscle on the back of the top half of your arm) with your other hand, and stretch it across the chest. Rest the arm you are stretching in the V (that is, elbow crease) of your other arm. Press both arms into the chest. Make sure that you keep the stretching arm straight. Repeat the same stretch exercise with the other arm.

Wrist and forearm stretch: Extend the right arm in front of you. With the left hand, go over the top of the hand of the extended right arm and gently press the fingertips downward to the floor. Repeat with the left arm.

Cardiovascular or aerobic fitness

Aerobic exercise strengthens your heart and lungs, and makes you feel less fatigued. Aim to do about 2½ hours (a total of 150 minutes) of moderate activity a week or at least 1½ hours (90) minutes of vigorous activity weekly. You can also have aerobic bursts of 10 minutes or more throughout your day.

Moderate activities include raking leaves, vacuuming, pushing a lawn mower, or playing with your children.

Vigorous activities include jogging in place, using a jump rope, or riding a stationary bike to the point that you are breathing harder.

60

Exercise equipment

You don't have to spend money to get and stay in shape, but there are some useful pieces of equipment you can buy to use at home if you think you will find it motivational. Some are more expensive than others, in which case be sure that you will use an item before investing, and also measure up to make sure you have adequate space.

- Treadmill
- Stationary bike
- Exercise DVDs
- Jump rope

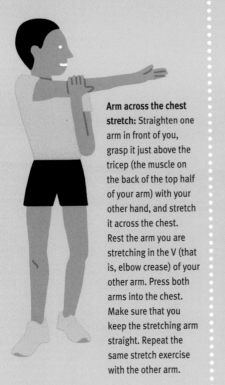

Jogging in place: Before you begin, make sure you feel balanced. Raise one leg so the foot is a few inches off the ground, then return the foot to the floor. At a fast pace, lift the other leg and then return the foot to the floor. Both feet should only be on the floor for a very short time. Visualize this activity as running in place at a slow pace. Relax your upper body, and bend your arms at the elbows so that they are in front of your body. As you raise one leg the opposite arm should be raised and move forward naturally. Do this as fast as you can without compromising your balance.

Jumping jacks: Stand with your arms straight down at your sides. Make sure your legs are straight and close together, knees slightly bent. Jump both legs out so they are wider than your shoulders while clapping your hands above your head in a smooth, rhythmical movement. If you are uncomfortable jumping, have your legs straight and close together, slightly bent knees, then extend one leg out to the side a little further than your shoulder. Quickly return the leg so the feet are together and repeat with the other leg. Do the same movements with the arms.

Muscular strength and endurance

When you are building stronger muscles, you are developing muscular fitness. If you are increasing how long you can use your muscles, you are developing muscular endurance. You can make muscles stronger by pushing or pulling against them. Try to do strengthening exercises two or more times a week. Focus on working the large groups (such as your arms, legs, back, chest, and core abdominals). You can gain muscular fitness by doing exercises like push-ups and leg lifts, or even by doing housework and yard work, such as scrubbing floors or pulling weeds.

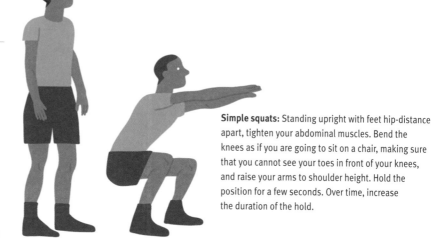

Simple squats: Standing upright with feet hip-distance apart, tighten your abdominal muscles. Bend the knees as if you are going to sit on a chair, making sure that you cannot see your toes in front of your knees, and raise your arms to shoulder height. Hold the position for a few seconds. Over time, increase the duration of the hold.

"Swim" on the floor: Place some kind of padding on the floor for comfort. Lay face down on the floor. Extend your arms straight in front of you, shoulder-width apart, but do not lock the elbows. Extend your legs straight behind you, hip-distance apart. The tops of your feet should be touching the floor. Tighten your abdominal muscles. Raise your right arm and your left foot while keeping your head facing the floor, in line with the spine. Lift your head, but do not tilt it back or forward. Hold the position for a few seconds. Repeat using the opposite arm and leg.

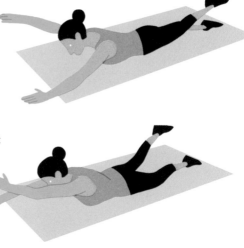

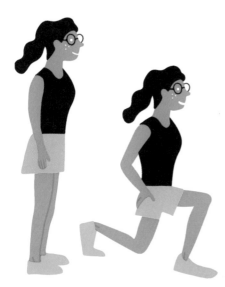

Lunges: Wear low-heeled shoes with traction, such as gym shoes. Before you begin, make sure you feel balanced. With both feet on the ground, hip-distance apart, raise one leg and step forward while still balanced. Bend your front knee as far as you can, making sure your back leg is straight and directly behind you, and that you're on the ball of the back foot. Place your hands on the front of your thigh for support. Make sure your front knee does not go beyond the toes—you may have to move your front foot forward. Alternate each leg. Start slow and increase the number of lunges over time.

Modified push-ups: Place some kind of padding (an exercise mat, towel, or blanket) on the floor to provide comfort and protect the knees. Lie face down, then get up on your knees and place your arms under your shoulders, shoulder-width apart. Your arms should be straight but not locked at the elbows. Separate the knees so they are under your hips and hip-distance apart. Contract your lower stomach muscles and slowly bend your arms, keeping the elbows close to your body, lowering your body toward the floor but between your hands. Use your upper body and abdominals to bring you back up to the starting position. Repeat as many times as you can.

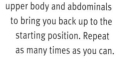

Check these out

www.webmd.com/fitness-exercise/guide/fitness-beginners-guide
A beginner's guide to exercise.

www.mayoclinic.com/health/fitness/HQ01543
Tips for staying motivated.

www.webmd.com/fitness-exercise/how-to-stay-active
How to stay active.

Do this...

✓ Make time for fitness: Schedule workouts in your calendar. Make exercise an "appointment" that you must keep. Take 10–15 minutes of computer or sitting breaks. Stand on one foot, stretch, or walk in place.

✓ Vary your workouts and make them fun and enjoyable. Identify three things you like to do and create a rotation schedule.

✓ Start exercise off with low- or moderate-intensity activities. Test yourself: can you talk or sing while doing the activity?

✓ Make rest and exercise a routine for health and fun.

...Not this

✗ Assume you will find some time to exercise; be inactive or sit by your TV or computer for more than two hours at a time.

✗ Get into an activity rut, doing the same things at the same times. You might become bored and give up.

✗ Do too much, too fast, too soon. Can't talk? Panting? In pain? Slow down!

✗ Exercise just to lose weight.

Household props

You may not know it yet, but there are already some useful props for stretching in your home. Consider the following:

Use a bed or desk as a simple prop to do stretches.

Use a chair or bench for stability to do dips.

Use resistance bands to help stretch and build strength and flexibility.

Simple core strengthener

This exercise can be done anywhere, anytime, so no excuses!

1 Bring your belly button back in toward your spine.

2 Hold this position for 5 to 10 seconds, then relax and repeat several times. Breathe normally and do not hold your breath while you are holding the position.

3 Repeat.

Beyond the home

It is most important that you find something that you really enjoy, because you will be more likely to stick to it. Exercising with others outside of the home can be motivational—taking up a team sport makes you accountable for showing up and adds a new social element to your life. Consider giving ballroom dancing or Zumba a try, or simply walk with a friend.

Keep a record

Logging the date, time, and type of exercise is a great idea. Making others aware of this new venture is also a great motivator—report to your chosen friend or family member every day. Hopefully they will be super-supportive, and be a source of encouragement.

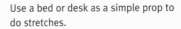
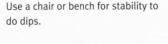
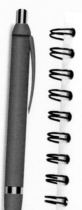

EXERCISE LOG

Monday: Fast walk, 40 minutes

Wednesday: 10 minutes on bike, 20 sit-ups. Stretches.

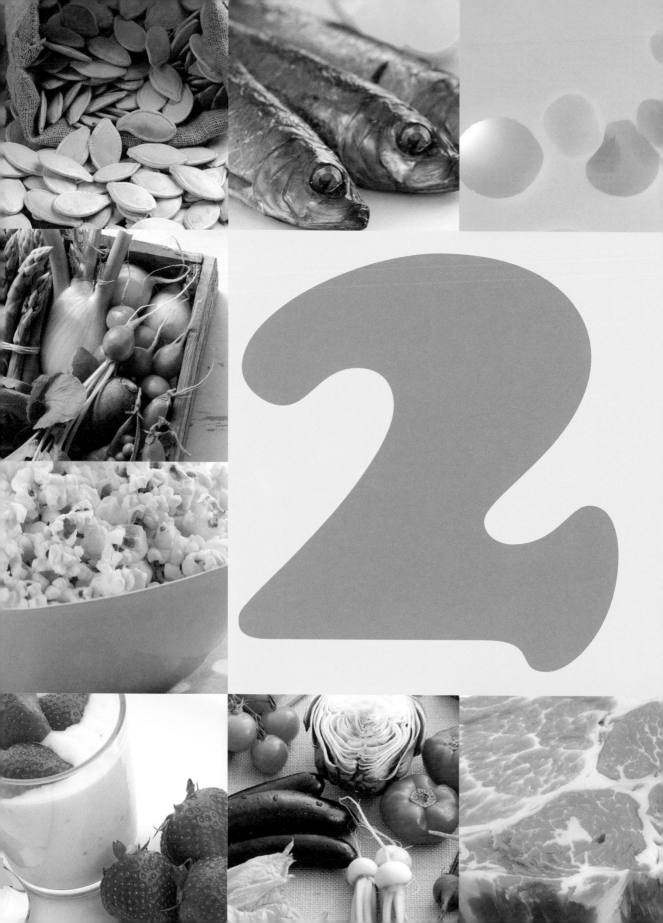

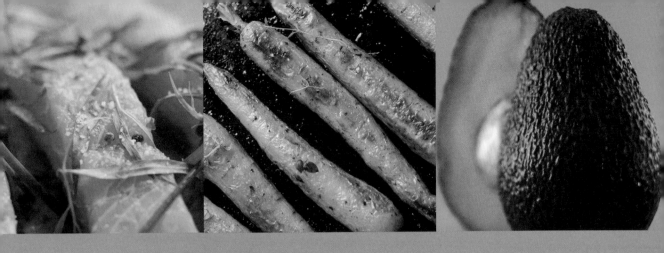

Out and about: Shopping

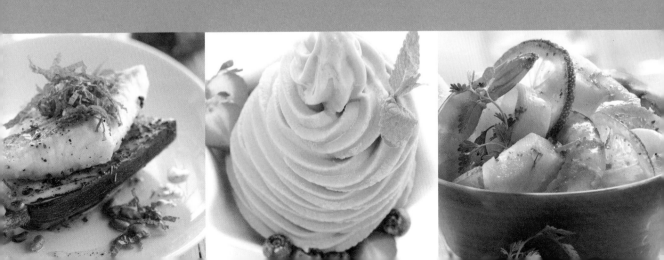

Shopping for health and flavor

A grocery store or market may seem like a maze, but with a good plan and a strategy you can save money while buying healthy and delicious food.

Where you shop and your shopping style will influence what you purchase and how much money and time you spend at the market. There are many types of food markets. Which do you frequent, and is your choice down to convenience or preference?

Convenience stores are plentiful but have a limited selection of snacks, pre-prepared items, and a few staples, usually at high prices. **Grocery stores** are larger and tend to cater to local community preferences, but may also carry some high prices. Some of these may be **ethnic stores** that specialize in particular foods. **Butchers' stores**, **bakeries**, and **fish markets** specialize in specific food items. **Farmers' markets** provide an array of locally produced fruits, vegetables, and other foods and trinkets, and support local economies. There is an increase in **gourmet food stores** that sell specialty and ethnic items, and charge prices that reflect their upscale nature. Then of course there are **supermarkets**, large chain stores stocking thousands of food products and household supplies. Recently there has been an increase in **wholesale markets**, where you become a member and shop for food in bulk.

Know your habits

You likely shop in several types of stores and switch between being a peripheral and a weaver type of shopper (see opposite). The key is to determine the strengths and pitfalls in your shopping style so that you can maximize your time and money while purchasing healthy foods you like and will eat.

If you prefer fresh fruits and vegetables and have time, shopping daily or several times a week can be pleasant and rewarding, especially if you can walk to the market.

However, if you are short on time, find healthy alternatives that allow you to shop less frequently. Frozen vegetables and fruits may be a more practical solution for you. Fresh and minimally processed foods are regarded as "more natural" and contain fewer secondary ingredients and additives. However, the term "processed" covers a broad range of items from a bag of pre-cut carrots to a loaf of bread to a frozen TV dinner. In general, the more processed a food is, the longer it may last. But compared to the fresh counterpart it will have more added ingredients and may cost more, although it may not appear that way. Think of a bag of frozen boiled potatoes, a box of dried mashed potato mix, or a bag of potato chips. How much "potato" was used to make those products, and how much does that cost compared to one potato?

None left? Is the pencil and notepad shopping list on your refrigerator or pantry door? Write it down before you forget.

 Do this...

✓ Check out the layout of the food market before you start shopping. Review what you need and "map out" your travel pattern for the shortest route to each section from where you need food.

✓ Shop after eating, so you can make decisions with your head and not your stomach!

 ...Not this

✗ Walk into the market without "mapping out" the organization and sections of the market. You are more likely to spend more time shopping and purchase things you do not need.

✗ Shop when hungry and veer toward high-calorie foods with low nutritional value. You will also be at your most vulnerable to supermarket marketing ploys (see pages 66–67).

Five money-saving tips

1 Create a shopping list based on staple foods and recipes for the week ahead.

2 Substitute items with in-store sales. Sometimes frozen or canned fruits or vegetables cost less.

3 Only buy in bulk if it is something you use frequently or does not spoil quickly.

4 Do not buy it just because you have a coupon.

5 Do you have a friend who grows their own veggies? Consider bartering or trading food, or join a cooperative.

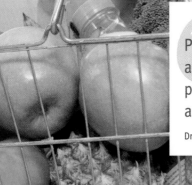

> Plan to shop around the perimeter of the store to save time and money. It is usually the shortest route to the dairy products, fruits and vegetables, breads, cereals, and grains and meat or meat substitutes sections of the market.

Dr. Claudia Sealey-Potts, Registered Dietitian/Nutritionist

Which type of supermarket shopper are you?

Peripheral shopper
"I hate doing this, am running through the major areas so get out of my way, I'm out of here." You run into the store, grab the items you think you need, and rush out. On the "pro" side, you may shop faster than most other people and spend less time at the market, but are you sure you are spending money effectively and selecting the best products for your needs?

Weaver shopper
"La de da, this is something that I can do for days and will take my time to complete." You weave through all the aisles and take time to look at many products and labels. On the "pro" side, you may be taking time to compare information regarding price, ingredients, and nutritional value. But are you buying unnecessary items and spending money on foods or things you really do not need or will not completely use?

Don't lose money on food waste

Three easy ways you can "lose money" on food. Imagine that on Tuesday you:

1 Buy a $3 cup of coffee at work. It sits on your office desk. At the end of the day you discard the leftover half. You threw away 50%, or $1.50 of your money.

2 Discard one third of a 10 lb (4.5 kg) bag of potatoes for which you paid $5.99 due to spoilage. You threw away 30%, or $2.00 of your money.

3 Buy 2 lb (900 g) of fish for dinner for five that cost $15.98. After dinner you notice you are discarding about 10 oz (280 g), an average waste of about 2 oz (55 g) per person. You threw away 32%, or $5.00.

That equates to a food waste loss of about $8.50 for the day. An average waste of that amount per day equals $3,103 per year.

Shopping for Meat, fish, and other proteins

Whether you are a meat eater or a vegetarian, protein is an important nutrient, and there are ways you can get the most for your money when buying this dietary staple.

What are meat and meat substitutes, and why are they important? The human body needs protein to grow and repair tissues and other body components. Protein, in turn, is made up of amino acids. Our bodies make some of these, but the ones the body does not make need to be obtained through the foods we eat. Some foods have all the amino acids you need—these are called foods with high-quality protein, or complete protein foods. In general, meats, poultry, fish, and dairy are complete protein foods. But luckily for vegetarians, there are also some plant-based foods that are complete protein foods. In addition, even if some foods are not complete proteins, by combining the foods wisely you can obtain all the complete proteins you need.

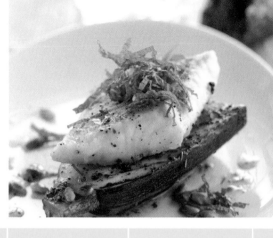

Fish provides both high-quality protein and healthy fats.

Eggs	Meats	Poultry
Eggs are the ultimate versatile food! Although you can get chicken, duck, and quail eggs, you probably only buy chicken eggs. Buy eggs and egg substitutes (which are egg whites) to eat as part of any quick meal or snack and in cooked or baked foods. Keep a couple of hard-cooked eggs in the refrigerator for a quick snack or as part of a meal, as in chopped in a main salad or a salad sandwich.	Although meats from sources such as pork or beef are high-quality proteins, they also contain fat. In some cases, they might even contain more calories from fat than they do from protein! So, when shopping, look for lean cuts of meat. This includes cuts such as bottom round steak, bottom round roast or steak, round tip roast, London broil, flank steak, sirloin tip side steak, and top sirloin steak. For pork, this includes tenderloin, loin roast, and top loin chops; and for lamb, lamb shank or loin chop.	Chicken, turkey, Cornish hens, guinea, duck, and goose are among the foods classified as poultry. You probably buy chicken and turkey most often. Keep it nutritious by removing the skin, which contains most of the fat. Turkey or chicken breast or drumsticks (without skin) are top poultry choices if you want protein and less saturated fat. But remember, a key for any poultry cut is to avoid or limit the skin, and to bake it instead of frying it.

70

Leaner meat

Look at the meat in the supermarket. Does it contain a lot of visible fat? Can you cut it out prior to cooking to cut back on fat? How much meat will be left?

Before you buy meat check for marbling (see right). That is the white fat globules or lakes of fat between the meat. It will help make the meat tender but add lots of fat to your diet. Skip the buy if there is a lot of marbling.

Lean cuts of meat need to be cooked correctly—avoid high heat or overcooking, which will make the meat tough. Cook using moist methods such as in stews.

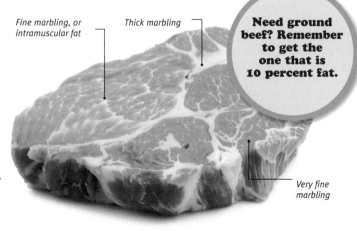

Fine marbling, or intramuscular fat

Thick marbling

Need ground beef? Remember to get the one that is 10 percent fat.

Very fine marbling

71

Buying fish?

Get a variety of both fatty and lean fish. Fatty fish such as salmon will give you some omega-3 oil, and lean fish, such as haddock, cod, or grouper, will be lower in fat.

 Do this...

✓ Buy high-protein, high-satiety snacks such as roasted soybeans or low-fat cheese sticks.

✓ Use two thirds creamy or coarse-ground mustard and one-third light mayo in your egg salad.

...Not this

✗ Buy bags of chips or candy for snacks.

✗ Use only regular mayonnaise in your egg salad.

PROTEIN COUNTER

BOILED BEANS | 1 CUP | PROTEIN

Lentils	8 g
Chickpeas	14 g
Pinto beans	15 g
Black beans	15 g
Navy beans	15 g
Pink beans	15 g
Black-eyed peas	16 g
White beans	17 g
Soybeans	22 g

Fish and seafood	Dairy	Vegetarian options	Nuts and seeds
When buying farmed fish and seafood, try species such as barramundi, catfish, clams, mussels, scallops, bass, tilapia, and trout. Other fish to buy are Pacific cod, Atlantic herring or sardines, wild pollock, wild salmon, and albacore tuna. If you like fish and buy and eat it regularly but vary it to get a range of nutrients, avoid species that are overfished.	Dairy products are a source of both high-quality protein and also calcium, so purchase these often. This allows you to double-dip your money for two major nutrients from one food group. Buy the best options: reduced-fat milk, fat-free yogurt (especially Greek-style yogurt), Cheddar, and low-fat cottage cheese. *With so many varieties to choose from, it's always possible to find a low-fat cheese that's big on flavor.*	If you are a vegan (see pages 102–103), beans—especially edamame—or soy products such as tofu, tofu crumbles, and soy milk are important foods to buy. Shop for staples such as dried and canned beans and nuts. Some grains, such as quinoa and buckwheat groat (kasha), can be important contributors to your daily protein intake. If you are a lacto vegetarian or a lacto-ovo vegetarian (eat dairy or eggs and dairy), these foods will provide high-quality protein, too.	Soy nuts, pumpkin seeds, peanuts, almonds, pistachios, and sunflower seeds are among the nuts highest in protein, so get these when buying high-protein snacks. However, watch the portion sizes as they are high in calories. 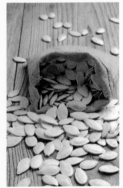

72

Ditch fat for protein

If used correctly, yogurt can be a versatile, low-fat source of protein. Try these two ideas for tasty treats:

• Instead of sour cream, buy Greek yogurt for a dip base. If you want a thicker spread, first strain the yogurt in a coffee filter for a few hours, before adding your seasonings.

• Mix cold vanilla-flavored yogurt and fruit juice in a tightly sealed container and shake. Increase protein by adding 1 tablespoon powdered skim milk.

73

Milky alternatives

Can't drink milk because of its side-effects? Buy the following:

• Low-lactose or lactose-free milks

• Aged cheeses

• Yogurts with no added milk or cream

All beans are good, so just buy the ones you like most whenever they are on sale. Use them for "Meatless Mondays."

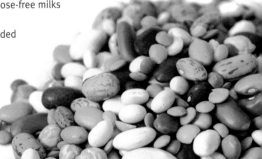

Shopping for Vegetables

"Eat your vegetables." You might have heard it from your Mom. Well, Mom's advice was wise. Start by buying smart!

Vegetables are naturally low in calories and high in essential nutrients. All vegetables contain some amount of potassium, folate, vitamin A, and vitamin C as well as compounds called phytonutrients. These compounds help keep your body working properly and many are antioxidants. Eating more vegetables as part of a healthy diet will not only help you control weight but also promote optimal health and help prevent serious health problems such as heart disease, type 2 diabetes, certain cancers, and high blood pressure. Due to their high water and fiber content, vegetables are a great choice for filling you up on fewer calories.

The usual recommendation for vegetables is about 5 servings, or 2½ cups, per day. It sounds like a lot, but it's easier than you think. If you have a large salad at lunch with a cup of a vegetable or tomato soup, and a cup of mixed vegetables and side salad at dinner, you can meet your daily recommendation.

You may wonder if it's better to eat vegetables fresh or cooked. In fact, all fresh, frozen, dried, and canned vegetables contain similar amounts of fiber and minerals, and cooking or drying vegetables does not destroy them. Vitamins that dissolve in fats, including vitamins A and E, are actually more concentrated in processed fruits and vegetables because the mild heat treatment makes the nutrients more available to your body. Cooking carrots or tomatoes can increase the level of phytonutrients available. On the other hand, heat used during the canning process—or the cooking of raw vegetables in water—can reduce the amount of B and C vitamins.

Save your vitamin C: Wrap fresh washed cauliflower, broccoli, or snap or green beans in plastic wrap and place in the microwave for 3–4 minutes. This quick, waterless cooking technique will help preserve the vitamin C in the vegetables.

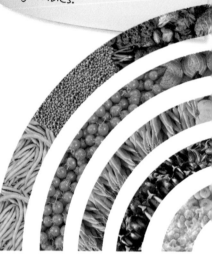

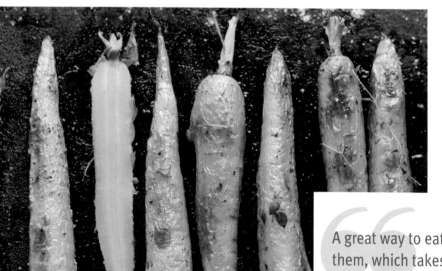

74

Perfectly tossed salad

Place all of your salad ingredients in a clean, unused plastic bag. Add a small amount of your favorite dressing. Toss around, and put in a bowl.

For a low-calorie dressing on fresh greens or cooked veggies, drizzle with a flavored vinegar.

> A great way to eat your veggies is to roast them, which takes away some of the bitterness. Add a dab of olive oil and seasoning.

Chelsey Millstone, Instructor and Nutrition Counselor

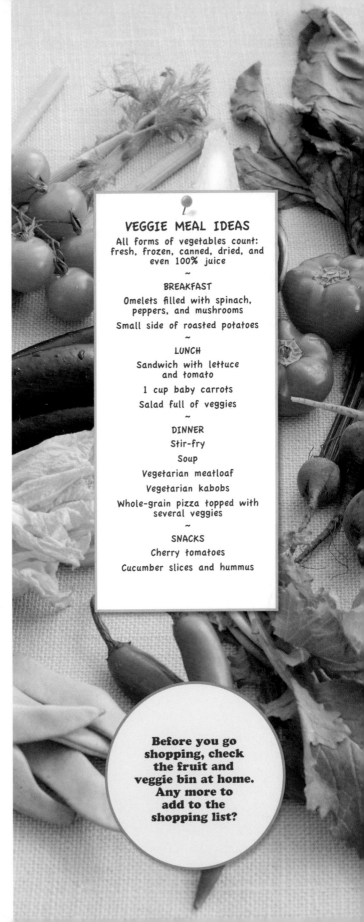

75

The right quality for the right use saves money

The nutritional value of vegetables will not vary hugely across brand and grade, but the shape, uniformity of color, and size will. If you are making pea soup, buy the less-expensive can or frozen bag of peas. Looks won't matter in a puréed bowl. Making a salad with peas as a centerpiece? Get the fancier ones, where shape, color, and uniform size will make for a beautiful dish.

76

Create a vegetable rainbow

A good way to eat more vegetables is to eat a variety of colored vegetables. Different colors of vegetables provide different natural phytonutrients that are good for your body and health. Choose vegetables that are green (such as dark leafy greens, broccoli, green pepper, green peas, and green beans), red (such as tomato, red pepper, and beet), orange/yellow (carrot, yellow pepper, pumpkin, squash, corn, sweet potato, and yam), purple/blue (eggplant and purple cabbage), and white (potato, cauliflower, onion, turnips, and white peas) to get a wide range and amount of phytonutrients.

77

Stock up your freezer

Many frozen vegetables are a great option because they can be found in their natural form in the freezer section of the grocery store. The advanced processing techniques used today minimize the exposure to time and temperature and prevent the loss of nutrients. Frozen vegetables are picked at the ideal time of peak ripeness and then quickly flash frozen to prevent spoilage and preserve nutrients.

78

In praise of the potato

A popular dieting trend has been to "avoid white things," including potatoes. While this may be a good principle for some foods, potatoes have nutritional value to offer for a relatively low number of calories and cost. Don't skip this economical and nutritious vegetable. Just include the skin and go easy with or skip toppings such as butter, sour cream, and bacon.

VEGGIE MEAL IDEAS

All forms of vegetables count: fresh, frozen, canned, dried, and even 100% juice

~

BREAKFAST
Omelets filled with spinach, peppers, and mushrooms
Small side of roasted potatoes

~

LUNCH
Sandwich with lettuce and tomato
1 cup baby carrots
Salad full of veggies

~

DINNER
Stir-fry
Soup
Vegetarian meatloaf
Vegetarian kabobs
Whole-grain pizza topped with several veggies

~

SNACKS
Cherry tomatoes
Cucumber slices and hummus

Before you go shopping, check the fruit and veggie bin at home. Any more to add to the shopping list?

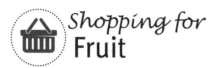

Shopping for Fruit

Fruits are as important as vegetables. So Mom's advice to eat more vegetables also applies to eating more fruit. You can buy and enjoy fruit in many forms.

Like vegetables, fruits are full of essential nutrients including vitamins, minerals, fiber, phytonutrients, and water. Fruit can help you maintain a healthy weight and reduce the risk of chronic diseases. Some people avoid fruit because it contains natural sugar. While the whole fruit is recommended over juices, natural sugar in whole fruit or 100% fruit juice is different from added sugars as it is accompanied by other health-promoting nutrients including fiber, vitamins, minerals, and phytonutrients.

The usual recommendation for fruits is about 4 servings (2 cups) each day. Together with vegetables, that's 9 servings per day. An easy way to meet this goal is to try to fill one half of your plate with vegetables and fruits.

When adding more fruits in your daily diet, try to buy them according to what's in season. This will help lower their cost and ensure peak flavor.
Spring: Apricots, pineapples, and strawberries.
Summer: Berries, cherries, grapes, peaches, plums, and watermelons.
Fall: Apples and pears.
Winter: Clementines, dates, grapefruit, kiwi, oranges, and tangerines.

Many fruits are available throughout the year, but the price will vary based on availability, and although quantity is important, eating a variety of fruits can better contribute to good health. Different fruits offer different nutrients, and eating a range will keep your tastebuds interested.

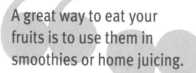

A great way to eat your fruits is to use them in smoothies or home juicing.

Jenna Braddock, Consultant and Sports Dietitian, University of North Florida

In the fridge right away:

Oranges, lemons, pineapples, berries, cherries, watermelons

Okay on the counter:

Bananas, cantaloupes, honeydews, pears, peaches, plums. (Refrigerate them if cut or they start to overripen and you do not plan to use them right away.)

79
Frozen and canned options
Many fruits can be found in their natural form, without added sugar or syrup, in the frozen food section of a grocery store. Frozen foods have been picked at the peak of ripeness and flash frozen to preserve nutrients.

Some canned fruit may have added sugar, in which case, drain and rinse the fruit to reduce sugar content, or choose fruit packed in water or 100% juice.

80
Create a fruit rainbow
Try to eat all the different colors of fruits to help create variety. Green is green grapes, kiwi, honeydew melon, and lime. Red is red grapes, cherries, cranberries, strawberries, and watermelon. Orange/yellow is apricot, cantaloupe, mango, orange, peach, and pineapple. Purple/blue is blackberries, blueberries, plums, and purple grapes. White is bananas, pear, and apples.

81
Bought too many?
Fresh fruit should never go to waste. If you think you've got more than you can eat, think ahead and take action to maximize your shopping:

Peel, cut into slices, wrap in plastic wrap, and freeze for a cooling treat.

Purée and mix with softened ice cream or yogurt. Put in the freezer and use later as a snack or dessert.

Make your own high-phytonutrient ice pops by half-filling a paper cup with grape, cranberry, pomegranate, or blueberry juice and sticking in a popsicle stick. Freeze and enjoy!

Once bought, store wisely

General rule: Use before the "use by" date on the package if one is included.

Fresh Use within a few days.

Frozen Store at 0°F (-17°C) or less and use within six months.

Canned Store at room temperature—most canned foods have a shelf life of two years.

Dried Store in a cool dry place—most will last from four months to a year.

Fruity fish
Fruit, especially citrus, can enhance the flavor—and appearance—of fish. Try slices or wedges of pineapple, lime, or orange in a shrimp salad, or a lime–orange sauce drizzled over fish.

FRUITY MEAL ENHANCERS

There is a variety of ways you can enjoy fruit any time of the year by using fresh, frozen, canned, or dried fruit, or 100% juice.

~

AT BREAKFAST

Top cereal or oatmeal with slices of bananas or peaches

Top pancakes with fresh berries

Drink a glass of 100% fruit juice

~

AT LUNCH

Eat fresh fruit for dessert

~

AT DINNER

Include orange sections or strawberries in a tossed salad

Add fruit like pineapple or peaches to kabobs

Add fruit to some meat dishes, like stir-fry chicken with pineapples or lamb tagine with prunes

Have fruit salad or poached apple or pear

~

AT SNACK TIME

Keep dried fruit in your work desk or bag

Mix fresh fruit with plain fat-free or low-fat yogurt

Stock up on dried fruit when on sale

Add raisins and/or unsweetened dried fruit to cereal, baked goods, and some meat or poultry dishes. Mix with peanut butter for your sandwich or have alone as a healthy snack.

 Do this...

✓ Choose whole fruits over fruit juices. This is the best way to enjoy their flavor and nutrients for the lowest amount of calories.

✓ Read the ingredients on juice cartons.

 ...Not this

✗ Drink cartons of fruit juice instead of eating whole fruits. When fruits are juiced, the fiber is removed, leaving sweet juice. It also takes a lot of whole fruit to produce a single serving of juice. This means that the calories in juice could be double or triple the amount in a single serving of whole fruit.

✗ Assume all fruit juice is healthy. Some blends contain concentrates, sugar, color, and flavoring.

Superfoods

Superfoods have exceptional nutritional qualities that both promote good health and help prevent disease. Here, we look at a handful of superfoods found in every grocery store, and a few more unusual ones.

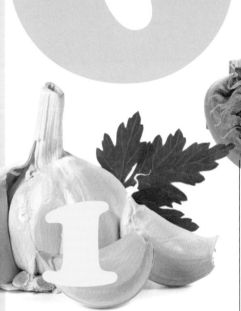

To avoid smelly garlic breath, chew fresh parsley, which neutralizes garlic odor— and is another superfood.

Garlic

What and why: Garlic is a bulb in the allium family, made up of a number of individual "cloves." Antibacterial, antifungal, antiviral, and an excellent general tonic, garlic is considered the king of the superfoods and has been found to be effective against a wide range of degenerative and infectious diseases, from cancer to the common cold.

How: Garlic is used as a flavoring in traditional cuisines around the world. It's most efficacious in its raw state, however, and even more so when it's crushed, chopped, or chewed to activate the sulfur compound allicin. The one downside to garlic is that it's famously antisocial, the odor lingering long and noticeably on the breath. Look out for fermented black garlic, which has no pungent odor but twice the antioxidants of white garlic and a far more mellow flavor.

As well as providing super nutrients, Romanesco broccoli looks super, too.

Cruciferous vegetables

What and why: Broccoli, kale, cabbage, cauliflower, Brussels sprouts, bok choy, arugula, watercress. Crucifers contain antioxidants, which protect healthy cells from damage caused by free radicals (toxic molecules), and are therefore associated with preventing the development of cancers and heart disease as well as other diseases linked to oxidative stress, such as diabetes, rheumatoid arthritis, and Alzheimer's. Each crucifer also has many other benefits—for example, kale is a rich source of iron, calcium, vitamin K (essential for blood-clotting and wound-healing), and lutein, which promotes eye health.

How: Cooking destroys valuable nutrients, so eat raw or do no more than lightly steam these invaluable veggies. It's important to chew thoroughly, as this helps form glucosinolates, the anticancer compounds. If you have a powerful blender, you can join the Green Smoothie movement—raw kale is especially good for this, blended with fruit such as orange, banana, or mango. The blender does all the chewing for you!

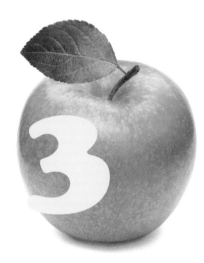

Eat apples with the skin on to benefit from all the nutrients.

Apple

What and why: An apple is a fruit—old-fashioned, pure, and simple. There's an old saying that an apple a day keeps the doctor away, and this still holds true. Apples contain pectin, which helps stabilize cholesterol levels and also binds to heavy metals such as lead and removes them from the body, which is helpful in our polluted modern environment. Apples also aid digestion and are therefore ideal accompaniments to fatty foods such as cheese or rich meats.

How: Choose organic apples where possible (or at least rinse non-organic apples), so that you can safely eat the skin, and eat them raw. It's best to eat an apple whole, chewing it well, but if you have digestive problems, grate it and eat it immediately. Apple juice is delicious but deprives you of the pectin-rich fiber.

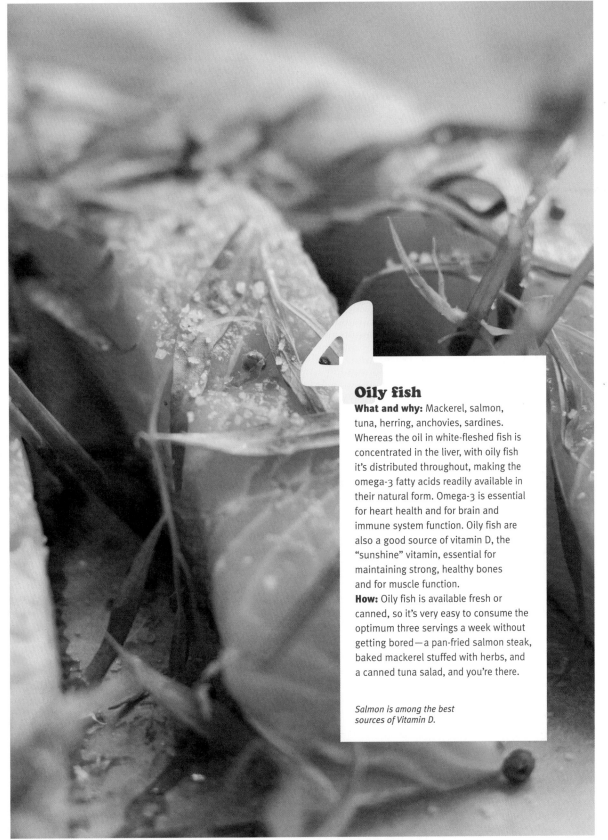

4

Oily fish

What and why: Mackerel, salmon, tuna, herring, anchovies, sardines. Whereas the oil in white-fleshed fish is concentrated in the liver, with oily fish it's distributed throughout, making the omega-3 fatty acids readily available in their natural form. Omega-3 is essential for heart health and for brain and immune system function. Oily fish are also a good source of vitamin D, the "sunshine" vitamin, essential for maintaining strong, healthy bones and for muscle function.

How: Oily fish is available fresh or canned, so it's very easy to consume the optimum three servings a week without getting bored—a pan-fried salmon steak, baked mackerel stuffed with herbs, and a canned tuna salad, and you're there.

Salmon is among the best sources of Vitamin D.

Continued next page

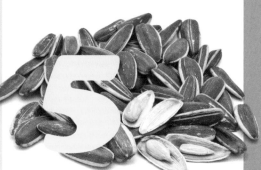

5

Seeds

What and why: Pumpkin, sunflower, sesame, flax, chia. An excellent source of protein and plant-based omega-3 fatty acids, seeds provide many other nutrients—they are, after all, literally the seed of a new plant—including important minerals such as magnesium, manganese, potassium, zinc, and copper. Seeds are anti-inflammatory and antioxidant and assist in hormone balance. Flax and chia seeds become mucilaginous when soaked in water and are excellent for maintaining a healthy digestive tract. Pumpkin-seed butter makes a good alternative to butter, and sunflower lecithin is a GMO-free alternative to soy lecithin as a nutritional supplement.

How: Pumpkin and sunflower seeds are an instant snack, but the nutrients are more bio-available if the seeds are first soaked in water and then dried in a very low oven. Sesame seeds are tiny, so sprinkle them on salads or oatmeal or make hummus or dressings from tahini. Unsoaked flax and chia seeds can also be sprinkled, but because they are so mucilaginous it's essential to drink plenty of water.

6

Avocado

What and why: Avocado is a fruit that's more usually used in a savory context than a sweet one. Anti-inflammatory and antioxidant, avocado is a good source of heart-healthy monounsaturated fat, promotes absorption of nutrients, and contains generous levels of fiber, potassium, and B vitamins.

How: Avocados are the ultimate healthy fast food—simply halve lengthwise and season with a little sea salt and freshly ground black pepper; blend into a guacamole dip; or crush onto crispbread and sprinkle with sunflower seeds. To make an instant superfood "ice cream," blend avocado with frozen apple slices; no sweetener required.

Use mashed avocado in place of mayo or butter in sandwiches.

New superfoods on the block

"New" superfoods are introduced on a regular basis, although usually their usefulness has been known to the local population for centuries. Those listed below are currently enjoying a high profile.

Name	Origin	What and why	How
Quinoa (keen-wah)	Andes	Tiny pseudo-cereal grain; contains all nine essential amino acids; gluten-free	Serve as a side instead of rice; add to soups; cool and use in salads
Goji berries	Himalayas	Bright red dried berries; contain B and E vitamins, minerals and carotenoids	Mix with pumpkin seeds for an instant snack or whiz them in smoothies and desserts
Moringa	Africa, Asia	Powdered leaves of the Moringa oleifera tree; high-protein, low-fat, and carbohydrate; rich source of vitamins and minerals	Blend into green smoothies or add to water or juice
Cacao powder	Amazon	Seed of Theobroma cacao ("cacao, the food of the gods"); good source of minerals, fiber and essential fatty acids; stimulates endorphin release	For optimal health benefits, add raw cacao powder to smoothies and raw desserts

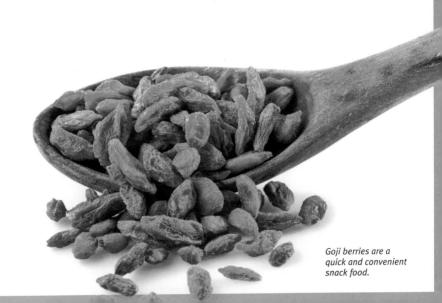

Goji berries are a quick and convenient snack food.

Shopping for
Fats and sweets

We all eat fats and sugars. The key is knowing which ones to buy, which ones to consume, and how much.

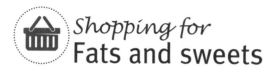

Fat-free, sugar-free, natural, or organic does not mean low-calorie. Read the label for calories per serving.

 ## Do this...

✓ Buy foods with zero trans fat.
✓ Buy foods with zero saturated fat.

...Not this

✗ Buy foods that have more than 1 gram of trans fat.
✗ Buy foods that have more than 5 grams of saturated fat per serving (try to eat less than about 20 grams in total per day).

Fats are bad! Sugar is bad! But we all eat them. How can we buy and eat them wisely?

Types of fat

There are visible fats and invisible fats. **Visible fats** include butter, margarine, oils, lard, hydrogenated fats, and cream cheese. **Invisible fats** are already in the foods you eat, so it is hard to know how much you are eating or to know if it is a healthy or an unhealthy fat. Common sources of invisible fats are whole milk, cheese, cakes, cookies, flaky pastries, some breads, pie crusts, cakes, pancake or waffle mixes, fried foods, donuts, some candies, chocolates, chips, packaged popcorn, or frozen foods.

From a chemical and nutrition perspective, monounsaturated fats have one double-bonded (unsaturated) carbon in the molecule. Polyunsaturated fats have more than one double-bonded carbon in the molecule. Both fats (which are actually oils) can help reduce bad cholesterol levels and risk for heart disease. Although all these fats have about the same number of calories, some are more important in health promotion (monounsaturated and polyunsaturated fats) than others (saturated fats, hydrogenated fats, lard, and trans fats). So it is important to read the ingredients label to know what type of fat is in the food, and to read the nutrition label to know how much you are getting in a serving.

Sugar and other sweeteners

Most people buy **granulated sugar**, which is sucrose. Did you know that confectioner's sugar is the same thing, just more finely ground? **Brown sugar** tends to contain more molasses than granulated sugar, but that does not mean it is less refined. In some cases, the granulated sugar (made by removing the top layer of molasses) has had molasses re-sprayed onto granulated sugar to make brown sugar. **High-fructose corn syrup**, or corn syrup, is used in many commercial foods. **Honey** is made by bees, and is essentially a mixture of sugars such as dextrose, levulose, fructose, and sucrose in a water solution. (Notice that chemically most sugars end in "ose"? Look for that on the label.) Some people prefer honey over granulated sugar because it is made "by nature."

Sugar substitutes include aspartame (blue packet), saccharin (pink packet), stevia (green packet), and sucralose (yellow packet). In commercial food processing, any one or any combination of these may be used. Other products may also be added (such as fiber) to provide some of the textural qualities found in sugar and needed in the food when a sugar substitute is used.

Fat and sugar provide flavor and important characteristics to food, such as browning or texture. But we tend to eat too much of both. So, by finding ways to cut, not totally eliminate, fat and sugar, you can enjoy their benefits in moderation.

Sweet nothings

Don't assume that brown sugar is healthier than white—both types are in fact very similar and have little nutritional value.

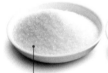 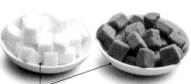

Granulated, the popular refined sugar—16 calories per tsp

Brown has a more robust flavor than granulated sugar due to the small amount of molasses—17 calories per tsp.

A convenient form of packing and serving sugar, a sugar cube is equal to a teaspoon measure.

What are omega-3 and omega-6?

Omega-3 and omega-6 are polyunsaturated essential fatty acids. In the body, omega-3 fatty acids are converted to important substances called EPA and DHA. Omega-3 fatty acids are found in cold-water fish such as salmon, sardines, herring, and mackerel. Walnuts and flaxseeds also contain EPA and DHA.

Vegetable or canola?

If the label says "vegetable oil," it is usually a combination of different oils. Although vegetable oil will cost less and can be used interchangeably with canola oil in recipes, buy the canola oil, which contains more omega-6 and omega-3, healthy fatty acids.

Superfish!

Sardines pack small in a can but are big nutritionally. They are a source of high-quality protein, healthy fats, calcium, vitamin D, and other nutrients. If canned, favor those packed in olive oil.

> Some quick-service restaurants now sell "snack items" such as wraps that are high in calories—so stick to fruit slices, small yogurt parfaits, or side salads with low- or no-calorie dressing.

Dr. Judith Rodriguez, Professor and Registered Dietitian, University of North Florida

5 easy ways to cut fats not flavor

1 Mix mashed cauliflower and chicken broth with your mashed potatoes, not butter.

2 Use applesauce and cinnamon or mashed bananas in your cake or muffin recipe instead of oil.

3 Use two egg whites instead of one egg for baking or your omelet recipe.

4 Use fat-free chicken, vegetable, or beef broth for your rice instead of water and oil.

5 Chill your soup or stew, then remove the fat layer on top before reheating and serving.

5 easy ways to cut sugar not flavor

1 Add a dash of lemon or lime, or a slice of fruit to cold sparkling water and enjoy in place of soda or fruit punch.

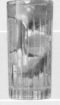

2 Top pancakes, waffles, or cereal with flavored yogurt or applesauce.

3 Replace one third of the sugar in recipes with sugar substitute.

4 Use ricotta cheese with flavored extract, or chopped or puréed fruit as your filling instead of jam.

5 Top a cake with an array of naturally sweet, naturally colorful fruit rather than sugary frosting.

Read all those labels!

The Ingredients List will inform you of the ingredients in descending order, by weight, if there is more than one ingredient. The Nutrition Facts panel provides information about the caloric value and nutrients in a serving of the food. For the true picture of the healthiness of the food you are buying, you will need to consult both lists. For example, sometimes manufacturers use a combination of sugars, so while "sugar" may not be listed as the first or top ingredient on a label, the cumulative use of these sugars will make the product high in sugars overall, in which case you'd be better informed by also looking at the Nutrition Facts label (see right).

Avoid saturated fats

Avoid fats that have cholesterol (from animal sources) or saturated fats, which may be naturally occurring or the result of processing. These include:

✗ Butter

✗ Coconut oil

✗ Fatback (pork fat)

✗ Hard margarine

✗ Hydrogenated fat (vegetable shortening)

✗ Lard

✗ Palm oil

Very important! If you eat more than the specified serving remember that you are getting more than is listed below.

Avoid foods with anything other than zero trans fats.

Nutrition Facts

Serving Size 1Tbsp (14g)

Amount Per Serving

Calories 80	Calories from Fat 80

	% Daily Values*
Total Fat 8g	**12%**
Saturated Fat 2.5g	**13%**
Trans Fat 0g	
Polyunsaturated Fat 3g	
Monounsaturated Fat 2.5g	
Cholesterol 0mg	**0%**
Sodium 85mg	**4%**
Total Carbohydrate 0g	**0%**
Dietary Fiber 0g	**0%**
Sugars 0g	
Protein 0g	**0%**

Vitamin A 15%	•	Vitamin D 15%
Vitamin E 15%	•	Vitamin B6 35%
Vitamin B12 20%		

*Percent Daily Values are based on a 2,000 calorie diet. Your Daily Values may be higher or lower depending on your calorie needs.

	Calories	2,000	2,500
Total Fat	Less than	65g	80g
Sat Fat	Less than	20g	25g
Cholesterol	Less than	300mg	300mg
Sodium	Less than	2400mg	2400mg
Total Carbohydrate		300g	375g
Dietary Fiber		25g	30g

Select foods that are a good source of fiber, 2.5–4.9 g per serving.

Look for high vitamin values (20% or above for at least one vitamin). Avoid foods with values of 5% or under, as these are considered to be low in vitamins.

Shop for healthy fats

Monounsaturated fats, buy:	Polyunsaturated fats, buy:
Canola oil	Corn oil
Olive oil	Soybean oil
Peanut oil	Safflower oil
Sunflower oil	
Sesame oil	

90

Make your own healthy spread

Don't want to give up the taste of butter? Mix one-third butter and two thirds canola oil. Put in the fridge and use (sparingly) as your soft spread.

91

Beware of "sugar-free"

Small candies or other products labeled "sugar-free" commonly have sugar substitutes known as sugar alcohols (which do not contain alcohol) and include erythritol, glycerol, isomalt, lactitol, maltitol, mannitol, sorbitol, and xylitol. Be careful—they are not calorie free, and eaten in large quantities may act as a laxative.

92

Lower in calories? Not really...

Honey is in a water solution so it is more concentrated. That's why it tastes better than sugar. You are getting more "sugar" and a few micronutrients per teaspoon.

Sugar: 16 calories per tsp

Honey: 21 calories per tsp, but use less than sugar for the same sweetness and fewer calories

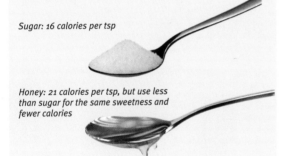

The difference between extra-virgin and regular olive oil is in the intensity of flavor—extra-virgin being the stronger.

Regular olive oil: 40 calories per tsp

Extra-virgin: 40 calories per tsp, but use less than regular oil for more flavor and fewer calories

93

What about plant stanols or plant sterols?

Some spreads contain plant stanols or plant sterols, which are substances found in plants. These substances are similar to cholesterol, but they work to help remove the harmful or "bad" cholesterol from the body.

Scanning the ingredients

Read the ingredients on the label (see below) to check if the spread you are buying contains stanols or sterols. These are "heart healthy" fats—but still be careful with the calorie intake by watching serving sizes.

INGREDIENTS: BUTTER (SWEET CREAM, SALT), **OIL BLEND (PALM FRUIT, CANOLA, PURIFIED FISH OILS),** WATER, CONTAINS LESS THAN 2% SALT, **PLANT STEROLS,** WHEY, SORBITAN ESTER OF VEGETABLE FATTY ACIDS, NATURAL FLAVOR, SUNFLOWER LECITHIN, VEGETABLE MONOGLYCERIDES, VITAMIN A PALMIATE, BETA-CAROTENE COLOR; LACTIC ACID, POTASSIUM SORBATE, TBHQ, CALCIUM DISODIUM EDTA

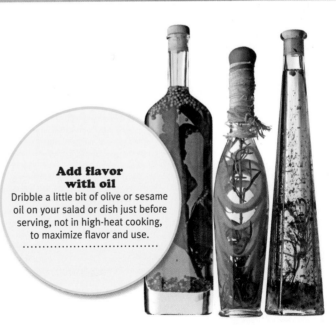

Add flavor with oil

Dribble a little bit of olive or sesame oil on your salad or dish just before serving, not in high-heat cooking, to maximize flavor and use.

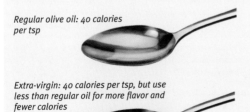

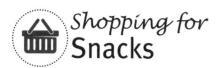

Shopping for Snacks

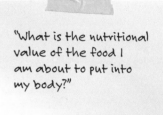

"What is the nutritional value of the food I am about to put into my body?"

The snack industry is a multi-billion dollar industry and new types of snacks are constantly introduced. By mastering a few shopping techniques, you can always figure out the best choice.

Snacks can be great way to stave off hunger and fill in some nutritional gaps. For adults, eating a snack can prevent you from becoming ravenously hungry and then overeating at the next meal. For children, eating a healthy snack can add much-needed nutrition. While it is better to make your own snacks, sometimes busy schedules do not allow this. You may be out of the house and suddenly find yourself hungry. The key to buying snacks is

that they should be nutritious and fulfilling so you can feel well and stay on track with your eating goals.

There are so many snack foods on the market that the choice can be overwhelming. However if you follow these simple guidelines, you will be able to make healthy snack choices whether you planned on buying snacks at the grocery store or you suddenly are in need of something quick to eat.

94

Look beyond the marketing

As with any snack, even supposedly healthy ones such as kale chips, hummus crackers, and baked chickpeas may sound appealing but may have additional fat, salt, and sugar added. As always, read the labels and favor those high in fiber with more than 20% of vitamins or iron.

95

How much is "healthy"?

So you know to pick snacks with little processing, fat, and sugar, but ones that are high in nutrients such as fiber and vitamins. But how does this translate to the amounts you see on the labels? Here are some key amounts to bear in mind to help you make quicky and healthy decisions:

> Get five plastic snack packs and fill with ½ cup dry cereal such as round oats or puffed rice and ½ cup raisins or other dried fruit and nuts. Pack for the office midday snack.

Judith C. Rodriguez, Professor, Nutrition and Dietetics

Calcium	
Iron	20% or more is considered to be a "rich source"
Vitamin A	
Vitamin C	
Fiber	5 g or more considered a "high source"
Fat	3 g or less considered "low fat"
Sodium	140 mg or less per serving considered "low-salt"
Sugar	Look for "no added sugar"

96

Be sure you only eat one serving

A store-bought snack bag often contains several servings. Not being aware of the number of servings leads to overconsumption of calories. You can always eat part of it and save the rest for later. And remember: If you don't buy it at all, you won't eat it!

20 Tasty snacks under 150 calories

Medium apple
3 inches/7.5 cm diameter,
6½ oz/182 g, 95 kcal

Blueberries
1 cup/148 g, 84 kcal

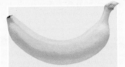

Medium banana
7 inches/18 cm long,
4 oz/118 g, 105 kcal

Dried apricots
4 halves, ½ oz/14 g,
136 kcal

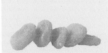

Raisins, seedless
1 oz/28 g (approx.
60 raisins), 85 kcal

Prunes, pitted
1½ oz/38 g (approx.
4 prunes), 91 kcal

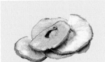

Dried apple rings
1½ oz/38 g, (approx.
6 rings), 93 kcal

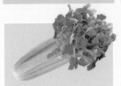

Celery
½ cup/50 g, 8 kcal

Tomatoes, grape
½ cup/79 g, 13 kcal

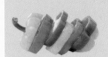

Peppers
Raw, sliced, 1 cup/92 g,
29 kcal

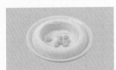

Hummus, home-prepared
3 tbsp/45 g, 81 kcal

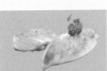

Chicken breast
Deli, rotisserie seasoned,
sliced, prepackaged,
approx. 3 slices, 1 oz/36 g,
36 kcal

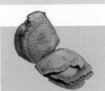

Roast beef
Separable lean and fat,
trimmed to ⅛ inch fat, all
grades, 2 oz/57 g, 124 kcal

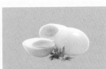

Large hard-cooked egg
2 oz/50 g, 78 kcal

Pistachio nuts
Dry roasted, no added salt,
½ oz/21 g (approx.
49 kernels), 121 kcal

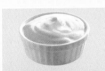

Greek yogurt
Plain, non-fat, 6 oz/170 g,
100 kcal

Cottage cheese
Reduced fat, 2% milk fat,
4 oz/113 g, 97 kcal

Milk, low-fat
1% milk fat, 8 fl oz/240 g,
102 kcal

Chocolate almond milk
Sweetened, ready to drink,
8 fl oz/240 g, 120 kcal

Frozen yogurt
Strawberry, 70 g, 80 kcal

Calorie, ingredient, and nutrient content may vary by brand.
Always read the Nutrition Facts label and the Ingredients List to verify ingredients, nutrient content, and calories per serving.

Calories and serving sizes

When shopping, it's helpful to know what is high and low in calories, as well as the recommended serving sizes—and weigh that up against how much you will actually eat.

> The more you know about the foods you routinely eat, the more you can tailor your choices to meet your calorie needs.

When shopping, you'll need to look at the number of calories in certain foods and, just as important, the serving size of prepared foods. Then determine how much you are likely to eat, to get a real account of the calories you will be taking in.

Foods that are high in calories, or calorie dense, tend to be high in fat and/or sugar:
• Casseroles
• Desserts
• Cream soups
• Certain cuts of meat or cheese, either alone or in combination with pasta, rice, or another starch

Foods that tend to be low in calories, or less calorie dense, are:
• Fruits and vegetables
• Low- or non-fat dairy products
• Whole grains

Keep your eye on the size
If buying frozen dinners, you need to look at the serving size to make sure you know how many calories you will eat. For cake mixes, you need to determine what other ingredients will be added. And some prepared items, such as salad dressings, give calories for small serving sizes, such as a tablespoon. So, always read the nutrition label for serving size and calories per serving, and make sure you know how big that serving really is.

Substitute lower-calorie items when possible. Being a calorie hunter will make you aware of places you can cut calories.

Visual guides for portion estimation
Keeping the visual guidelines below in mind will help you quickly estimate how much of a food you are eating and therefore control portions and calories to be able to determine how much to purchase.

Hand measure	Equivalent	Foods
	An average-size fist = 1 cup	Salads, whole or cut-up fruit and vegetables, cooked beans, cooked or dry cereal, cooked pasta, rice or other grains
	Your palm = 3 oz (85 g)	Cooked meat, poultry, seafood
	A small cupped handful = 1 oz (30 g)	Nuts, seeds, dried fruit
	A large cupped handful = 2 oz (55 g)	Dry snacks, i.e. pretzels
	Your thumb (from tip to base) = 1 oz (30 g)	Cheese
	Your thumb tip (from tip to first joint) = 1 tablespoon	Peanut butter, hummus, sour cream, salad dressing
	Your fingertip (from tip to first joint) = 1 teaspoon	Butter, margarine, mayonnaise

98

Three easy ways to cut calories from your food shop

1 **Buy in small amounts** or put back anything you are tempted to eat in excess.

2 **Look for lower-calorie substitutes** for items you usually buy and pick those instead.

3 **Walk around one more time** before going to the checkout and put back some of the "naughtier" or unnecessary items.

 99

Don't be fooled!

Look at the serving size. Imagine two 12-oz (340-g) packages of lasagna. A quick glance at "calories" on the label shows 400 calories for Lasagna A and 500 for Lasagna B. Careful inspection shows a serving size for Lasagna A is 4 oz (110 g) but a serving size for Lasagna B is 6 oz (170 g). Lasagna B is actually lower in calories overall, and probably is a more realistic serving size.

> **Love those creamy mashed sweet or white potatoes? Use undiluted evaporated low-fat milk instead of butter to decrease fat and increase calcium.**
>
> Dr. Judith C. Rodriguez, Professor and Dietitian, University of North Florida

 100

Portion size illusion

Notice how the portions look smaller when the plate or bowl is larger. To make the illusion work in your favor and help prevent overeating, go back to your grandmother's crockery or source some vintage plates.

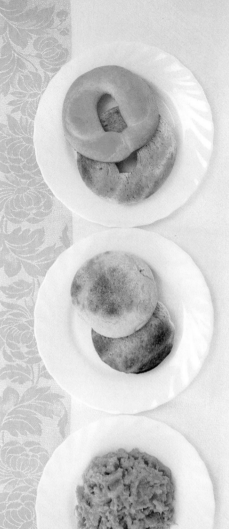

CALORIE COMPARISONS

SIZE MATTERS:

Bagel, 3 inches (7.5 cm) | **140 calories**

Bagel, 6 inches (15 cm) | **350 calories**

TOPPING MATTERS:

English muffin | **140 calories**

English muffin with 1 tsp each butter and jelly | **249 calories**

INGREDIENTS MATTER:

Baked sweet potato, mashed, 1 cup | **114 calories**

Sweet potato casserole, 1 cup | **236 calories**

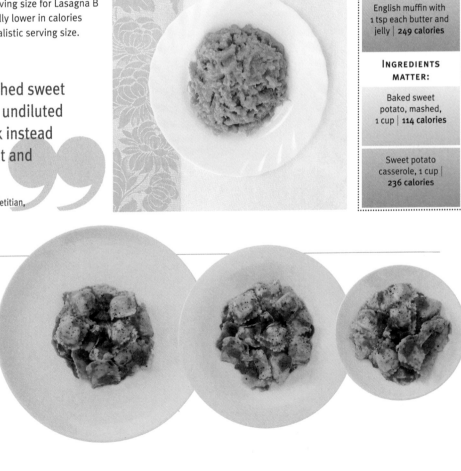

Be ingredient savvy

Maintaining healthy eating habits requires watchfulness and a keen sense of the types of ingredients in the foods you buy and eat.

It is not sufficient to just look at the pictures on the food packages or to assume that you are purchasing high-quality, nutritious food because it comes from a respectable grocery store or well-known manufacturer. With many foods consumed on the go and purchased in packaged, ready-to-eat, or convenient forms, the Ingredients List is the key to making wise and healthy food choices.

Many convenience or packaged foods contain lots of ingredients that are difficult for consumers to pronounce, or understand. Most of these ingredients seem to have been created in a food science lab. It is also important to note that some of the claims on packages require further investigation and can only be verified by reading the Ingredients List. One example: A food package may claim that there is "no trans fat"; however, if you read the ingredient list you may find that one of the ingredients listed is partially hydrogenated oil, a source of trans fat.

Resist seduction!

Grocery shopping can be overwhelming for even the most experienced shoppers, and a consumer trend toward purchasing more "natural" foods has forced marketers to create seductive labels that have added to the confusion. With all of the marketing and advertising tactics used, it is hard to ascertain what is really inside your food. You may come across foods that are labeled "natural," "healthy," or "organic" to entice you to pick the product. Always look beyond clever packaging and select truly nutritious and wholesome foods.

Preservatives

Some food ingredients are added by companies to help preserve the food items. These ingredients may help improve the taste and texture of the products. At times additional ingredients may contribute excessive intakes of calories, fat, sugar, and salt, thereby making the food item less desirable as a healthy option.

"Real," fresh foods should contain no hidden ingredients. Buy as many as you will manage to eat or store before they perish.

broccoli	$3.49
asparagus	$2.99
onions	$3.59
apples	$3.99
strawberries	$4.29
bananas	$2.58
grape juice	$5.39
low-fat milk	$3.99
evaporated milk	$1.09
Cheddar cheese	$6.99
low-fat yogurt	$1.19
chicken breasts	$5.99
can tuna	$1.19
large eggs	$2.19
can chickpeas	$1.19
fettuccini	$1.59
parboiled rice	$5.99
French bread	$2.39
whole wheat bread	$3.59
ice cream	$3.79
potato chips	$3.29
Milano cookies	$3.59
diet cola	$4.00
gum	$1.29
frozen peas	$1.79
dry roasted peanuts	$3.99
malt vinegar	$1.65
ginger tea	$2.79
tomatoes	$2.37
low-sodium ham	$4.99
mandarin oranges	$5.99
apple crumb pie	$4.49
salad mix	$3.69
cream soda	$1.00
English muffins	$4.19

Buy plentiful supplies for vitamins and fiber—a superfood!

Make the most of seasonal fruit, for variety throughout the year and top-level nutrition

Nutritious—with calcium and protein—and versatile for cooking

A kitchen staple and a source of protein and vitamins

Treats like this are packed with additives and preservatives—limit them to one per grocery shop

Check no salt has been added; rinse well before using if it has

Fewer calories, but beware the processed ingredients

Aids digestion. Try making your own from ginger root

Healthy fats; replace with peanuts in the shell for less salt

Needless sugar and calories—save money and ditch this!

 101

Running order

Ingredients lists are a hands-on way to know exactly what is in the food you are planning to consume. To do so you must note that ingredients are listed on the package in downward order of prevalence. This means that the first ingredient in the package makes up the highest proportion of the ingredients in that food item. It is also important to note that the first three ingredients are the ones that should matter the most to you.

 Do this...

✓ Use all-natural peanut butter, without added sugars and fat. In addition, natural peanut butter is often lower in sodium than the regular alternative.

...Not this

✗ Many brands of peanut butter contain added sugar and hydrogenated oils. These ingredients may change the texture of the final product, but do not have a major impact on flavor.

Quick-glance guide to additives and preservatives

Use the chart below to familiarize yourself with some of the more commonly used extra ingredients that food manufacturers add to their products, so that you will recognize them on food labels.

Give food body, stability, firmness, and/or texture	Enhance flavor	Add color	Make food last longer—common preservatives
Calcium chloride	Autolyzed yeast extract	Annatto extract (yellow)	Ascorbic acid (vitamin C)
Calcium lactate	Hydrolyzed soy protein	Beta-carotene (yellow to orange)	BHA
Carrageenan	Disodium guanylate or inosinate (notice the sodium!)	Caramel (yellow to tan)	BHT
Egg yolks	Monosodium glutamate, or MSG (notice the sodium!)	Dehydrated beets (bluish-red to brown)	Calcium propionate
Gelatin	Salt or sodium chloride	FD&C Blue Nos. 1 and 2	Calcium sorbate
Guar gum	Citric acid	FD&C Citrus Red No. 2	Citric acid
Mono- and diglycerides	Acetic acid	FD&C Green No. 3	Potassium sorbate
Pectin	Sodium citrate	FD&C Orange B	EDTA
Polysorbates	Guanosine monophosphate	FD&C Red Nos. 3 and 40	Potassium sorbate
Sorbitan monostearate	Inosine monophosphate	FD&C Yellow Nos. 5 and 6	Sodium benzoate (notice the sodium!)
Soy lecithin	Neotame	Grape skin extract (red, green)	Sodium erythorbate (notice the sodium!)
Whey	Quinine	Ferrous gluconate	Sodium nitrite (notice the sodium!)
Xanthan gum	Stearic acic	Sodium nitrite or nitrate	Tocopherols (vitamin E)

Want to avoid additives?

Shop for your groceries in the following order:

1 Fresh fruits, vegetables, frozen fruits and vegetables, fresh meats, dry beans, and plain roasted nuts.

2 Low-fat dairy, canned foods (drain and rinse to remove added salt or sugar), rice, pasta, and bread.

3 Rarely buy pre-prepared commercial mixes, frozen dinners, cured meats, snack foods, and baked items.

Simple guidelines for savvy shoppers

Follow these suggestions and you should be able to navigate the challenging environment of snazzy packaging and enthusiastic marketing.

Look for foods with only one or a few ingredients. These products will have gone through minimal amounts of processing.

Look for products featuring the word "whole," as in whole-grain breakfast cereals, crackers, pasta, and breads in your packaged food items, instead of refined grains.

Be mindful of added ingredients such as sugar, salt or sodium, and fat. Limit these wherever possible to maintain your healthy eating habits.

Unmasking marketing

Sensational and promotional language and enticing terms can lure the unwary shopper to buy unhealthy "healthy" foods.

Sometimes it seems that the harder we try to choose the healthy option, the more we're thwarted by marketing and advertising strategies that lure us toward unhealthy foods. However, with practice and armed with a few clues, it's easy to see beyond the marketing smokescreen.

No added sugar

This alluring label means that a product contains no sweetener, right? Wrong! It simply means that there is no added natural sugar—that is, the sort derived from sugar cane or sugar beet (sucrose). The product might, however, contain any one of several alternative sweeteners, especially high fructose corn syrup (sweeter and cheaper than "real" sugar) or sugar substitutes, as well as a whole range of other additives. Remember to check all labels for sugar and sugar substitutes, because they're used in the most unlikely products.

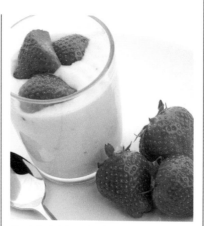

Check the labels on low fat and flavored yogurts for added sugar and other ingredients.

Low-fat

When a dairy product declares itself to be low-fat, that's what it will be. However, fat is where all the flavor is, so in order to make the product palatable, it is usually laden with sugar and possibly other additives instead, which are required to thicken and stabilize the base product. Be particularly wary of those fruit-flavored low-fat yogurts, which sound like the perfect snack food or dessert but have so much added sugar, starches, stabilizers, or flavorings that for your health's sake, you'd be better off adding fresh fruit to a full-fat yogurt.

Only 99 calories

This must be a winner, surely! Not so. There are calories and calories, and to be healthy you should always aim to get your calories from the healthiest source. With this in mind, beware—those low-calorie products are usually packed full of unnecessary additional ingredients. Cereal bars are particular culprits, luring you not only with the promise of low calories but with the magic words "whole grain," which also aim to convince you of the bar's value to your health. Look out for high levels of sweetener (any type), fats, artificial flavors, additives, and preservatives—if it takes you longer than a couple of seconds to read the Ingredients List, give the product a wide berth.

Organic

Manufactured products marked "organic" are not necessarily 100% organic or free of added chemicals—they might contain a mix of organic and non-organic ingredients, so if this is important to you, check the label, where the organic ingredients will be identified. When it comes to buying fruit and vegetables, consider freshness and food miles and decide whether it's better to buy a non-organic product grown locally or an organic product flown hundreds of miles before it reaches your table.

Always check labels for ingredients that are minimally processed, are in a whole or as a natural state as possible, and leave highly processed products on the grocery-store shelf.

A simple rule to follow, but an effective one!

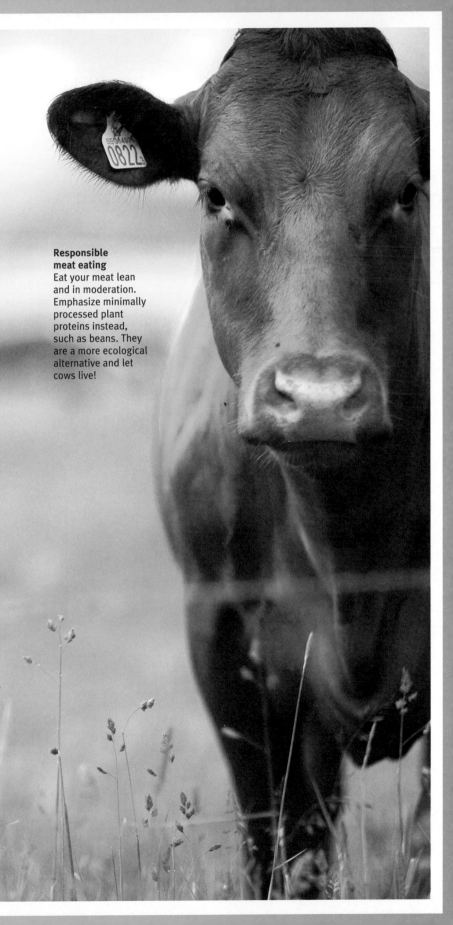

Grass-fed beef

The healthiest beef comes from animals raised on organic pasture, but for meat that is rich in essential fatty acids (EFAs), especially omega-3, and low in saturated fat, it must be grass-fed until slaughter. However, it's very common for animals to be grass-fed for a few months only, then "finished" on cereals, greatly reducing the levels of EFAs while raising the saturated fats. To be sure that the beef and other grass-fed meat you buy is most beneficial to your health, look for a reliable local producer—otherwise you might be paying grass-fed prices for cereal-fed meat.

Responsible meat eating
Eat your meat lean and in moderation. Emphasize minimally processed plant proteins instead, such as beans. They are a more ecological alternative and let cows live!

MSG

Monosodium glutamate (MSG) is a naturally occurring chemical, identified in the early 20th century by a Japanese chemistry professor, Kikunae Ikeda, as a component of seaweed and various other foods such as Parmesan cheese, tomatoes, and mushrooms. It creates the taste sensation now known as "umami," and it makes your taste buds very happy. So what's the problem with it? Simply this: It is added to manufactured products that we should eat in moderation, such as potato chips, encouraging us to eat more of them. And because it's been subject to some bad press, MSG is labeled under a number of other names, such as autolyzed yeast extract, calcium caseinate, and names containing "glut"— monopotassium glutamate, glutamic acid. For the sake of your health, get your umami kick from "real" foods!

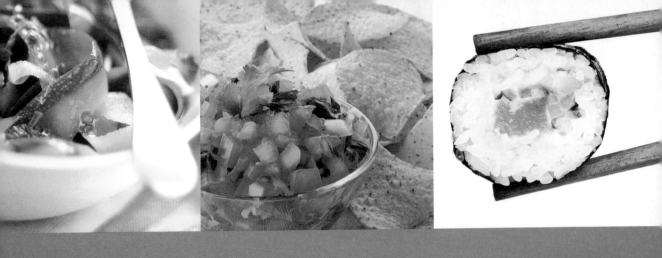

Out and about:
Restaurants and parties

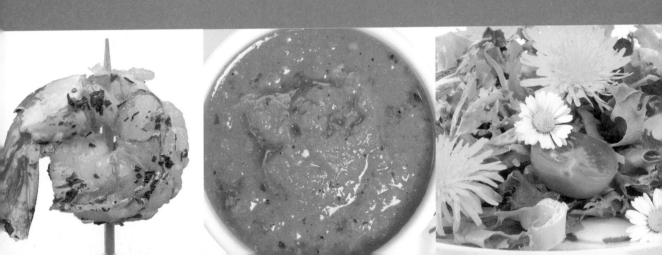

Healthy choices when eating out

Eating out provides a wide range of choice. The key is selecting eateries and foods that fit your time, lifestyle, and health goals while staying within your budget.

People are eating out more for many reasons. These may include changes in lifestyle, such as working families, lack of time, the increased availability and access to eateries, or a lack of cooking skills. There is also an interest in trying new foods, so people are going out to enjoy ethnic dishes. No matter where you choose to eat, you want food that is "priced right," and good-tasting and healthy options that make you feel satisfied about your eating out choices.

Popular eating out trends include:
• Selecting local meats, seafood, and produce
• Supporting eateries that have their own gardens for growing produce
• Selecting foods that are considered "safe" (prepared hygienically, not linked to any recent food scares, free from unknown ingredients that may provoke allergies, sourced responsibly)
• Buying gluten-free foods
• Selecting healthy meals and beverages for children
• Trying non-traditional or unfamiliar foods
• Selecting more whole grains

When you are trying to decide what to select from a menu, and how much emphasis to put on making healthy choices, consider how often you eat out. If it's more than twice a week, knowing how to make healthy choices becomes very important. If you rarely eat out and tend to eat well at home, a treat at a restaurant may not be a bad thing.

Watch your wallet, and your waistline
Eating out may seem easier than cooking food at home, but it can be costly. No matter what your income level, if you eat out, you may be spending the largest amount of your food budget on food away from home. Be careful; if you eat out frequently, just 25% of your meals eaten out can take up 40–50% of your food budget. Eating out may also lead to overeating.

If eating out often is part of your lifestyle, it is important to develop a system that helps cut food costs and enables you to select healthy foods. Like many people who work or lead busy lives, you may not have the time to go home for lunch, prepare food for lunch, or have facilities at work where you can keep your lunch. Furthermore, after a long day at work, you may prefer going somewhere to eat instead of cooking at home.

No matter where you choose to eat, you can make eating out healthily a choice, not a chance.

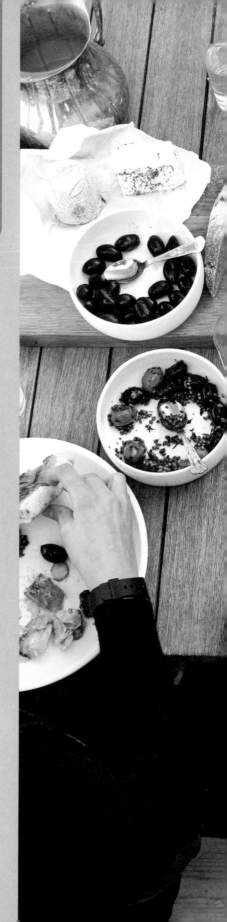

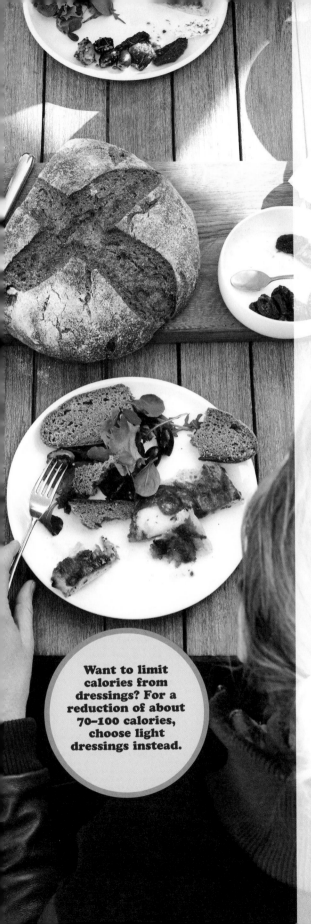

How often do you eat out?

Calculate how many times a week you eat out or eat take-out food. Is it more than 20% of the time? If so, take action to make eating out healthy. For example:

3 meals + 2 snacks x 7 days a week = 35 food events a week
1 meal + 1 snack as "eat out" activities x 7 days a week =
14 "eat out" events a week

That is **40%** of food events that involve eating out (14 divided by 35 = 40%). It's time to check the cost and nutritional contribution of these activities!

Don't overeat

Portion control is critical when eating out. When food is delicious and plentiful, it is very easy to overeat. To avoid this, use a smaller plate (your side plate, for example), or ask the waitress/waiter to box up half of your food to enjoy at home the next day.

Enjoy yourself, sensibly

If you're out with a group and fancy a drink, why not start with a glass of sparkling Prosecco instead of wine? At just 69 calories per glass, Prosecco is lower in calories than both red and white wine (125 and 122 calories per glass). Also, ordering by the glass is one way to think twice before drinking more, because it's easier to keep track; sharing bottles between groups often results in over-drinking. See pages 86–87 for more advice on limiting your alcohol intake.

Want to limit calories from dressings? For a reduction of about 70–100 calories, choose light dressings instead.

Do this...

✓ Go onto the website or get a calorie card or handout from your favorite eatery, then create a calorie budget such as "every meal will be 600 calories or less" and carry this with you.

✓ Have an appetizer as a main meal.

...Not this

✗ Rely on your instincts about what might be high or low in calories and order based on this.

✗ Eat bread and butter or appetizers before the meal.

Healthy eating at quick-service restaurants

It is unrealistic to decide to totally give up eating at QSRs. So the key is to make informed decisions about what you eat.

The hurried life that is emerging worldwide is fueling the use of quick-service restaurants (commonly referred to as QSRs), or fast-food restaurants. What makes QSRs so popular?

• They make food available quickly: You can get your meal in a few minutes, with little or no wait.
• They are relatively inexpensive: Compared to more formal eateries, the prices are generally lower for similar foods.

• They serve familiar and popular items: You usually know what they serve anywhere you go, especially if they are popular chain restaurants.
• They have standardized processes: There is consistency of experience in ordering, payment, and serving, and procedures tend to be the same everywhere you go.

There are some foods that are especially popular choices at QSRs. These include French fries, burgers, pizza, fried chicken, grilled chicken, tacos, burritos, hot dogs or bratwursts, ice cream, sundaes, bagels, baked potatoes, fried fish, coffee, and kebabs.

The common critique about QSRs is that the food is high in calories, fat, and salt or sodium. But many of these eateries have healthier alternatives that you can select, provided you are aware of them.

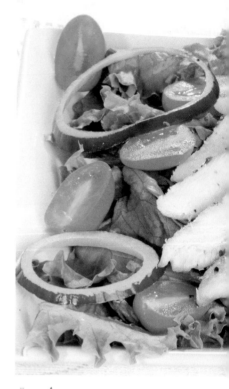

> **A large soda can add anywhere from 150 to 555 calories, depending on the size.**

107

Check in advance
Look up the QSR's website, have a read through the menu, and plan two possible healthy meals you could have there before going out to eat. By thinking of two, you have a backup if you change your mind or something's not available.

TOP 10 CALORIE CUTTERS

1
Breakfast sandwiches Ask for plain rolls or whole-wheat bread instead of croissants or flaky biscuits; Canadian bacon instead of bacon or sausage.

2
Hot cereals Opt for plain oatmeal. Add milk instead of cream, and sugar substitute or cinnamon instead of sugar. Skip the nuts and raisins to save a few calories.

3
French fries Ask for a small portion or share with a friend, or replace with a side salad.

4
Burger Order the regular size, plain, or with lettuce and tomato. Drop all the "creamy fixings." Do you dare to do half the bun?

5
Fried chicken Get grilled chicken instead, which is also among the top fast foods.

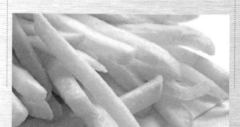

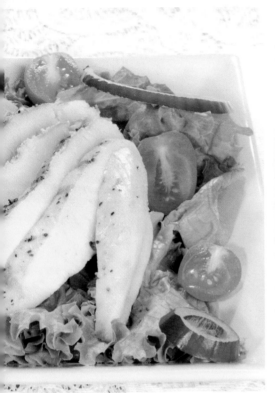

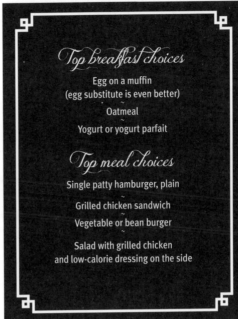

Top breakfast choices

Egg on a muffin
(egg substitute is even better)
~
Oatmeal
~
Yogurt or yogurt parfait

Top meal choices

Single patty hamburger, plain
~
Grilled chicken sandwich
~
Vegetable or bean burger
~
Salad with grilled chicken
and low-calorie dressing on the side

Make sure your salad is healthy
Salads with chicken can be a healthy, low-calorie, widely available choice when eating out, but make sure the chicken is grilled, not fried, and that you are careful with your choice and amount of dressing.

 108

Slow down
Just because it is called a fast-food restaurant, and you get the food fast, this does not mean you have to eat it fast. Take time to savor the food so you focus on quality, not quantity. You might find that you go off some of your favorite QSRs or dishes in favor of healthier, tastier options.

CALORIE COMPARISONS

PIZZA | CALORIES

Thin-crust cheese pizza slice | **230 calories**

Thick-crust cheese pizza slice | **312 calories**

HAMBURGER | CALORIES

Regular patty hamburger; single, plain | **232 calories**

Double regular patty hamburger with condiments | **575 calories**

FRENCH FRIES | CALORIES

French fries, 1 small serving | **323 calories**

French fries, 1 large serving | **497 calories**

6
Taco Order a soft corn taco, add lots of salsa, and skip the sour cream. Gotta guacamole? Only a small dab.

7
Hot dog Ask for the regular-size hot dog, add mustard or ketchup, and skip the other toppings. Do you dare to do half the bun?

8
Lemonade Ask for water and a few wedges of lemon instead. Squirt lemon juice into the water. Add your own calorie-free sweetener if desired, and you have your own, healthy lemonade, with added vitamin C!

9
Dressings and sauces There's no way round these—omit or, at the very least, limit all trimmings such as dressings, sour cream, mayonnaise, and ketchup.

10
Pizza Opt for thin crust with a vegetable topping. Avoid stuffed crusts and pizzas dripping in greasy cheese. If the pizza is large, take home half of it and eat it for lunch or dinner the next day.

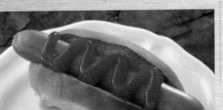

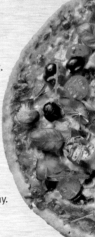

Healthy dining at restaurants

By eating out more, you become familiar with different foods. But, how do you know if your menu choice is healthy, or how it can be made into a healthier one?

No matter which country's cuisine you choose to sample, the main watchpoints for dining away from home remain the same:
• Saturated fat, salt, and sugar levels are harder to monitor when you haven't cooked the food yourself.
• You can easily end up eating more than you would have done by serving your own portions.
• The temptation to throw caution to the wind and ignore your healthy eating practices can be hard to resist when faced with a delicious and plentiful array of food and when surrounded by people who may not be dining out with the same health concerns as you.

But forearmed with a few key strategies and some background knowledge of the cuisine and the type of foods likely to be on offer, you can easily stick to your principles while enjoying the benefits of dining out. Afterall, even healthy people need a social life!

 (109)

Nourishing food for the soul

African-American cuisine, commonly known as "soul food," is a comfort to all, with its hearty meals full of flavor and great-tasting desserts. Traditional soul food tends to be high in sugar, fat, and salt due to the cooking methods and sauces/gravies used. But, there are ways to enjoy some popular dishes without losing touch with nutrition.

Choose vegetables—one of the great aspects of soul food is that there are so many great and tasty vegetables to choose from, such as okra and green beans.

Opt for collard greens instead of candied yams. Collard greens prepared without additional fat are low in calories (70 calories per cup) and fat and are a great source of vitamins A, C, and K, but candied yams (206 calories per cup) are often prepared with an abundance of sugar and fats.

If having meat, stick with grilled, baked, or broiled lean meats such as poultry and fish. Choose entrées such as grilled chicken breast or baked turkey wings to ensure that you are not ordering meat that is high in fats and calories.

Consider beans for your portion of protein, since they are a great source of this nutrition group but have much less fat and cholesterol compared to meat. Choose from field peas, black-eyed peas, lima beans and great northern beans, among others.

Watch out for foods that use words such as "creamy," "fried," or "smothered." Although tasty, these foods tend to be higher in fats and calories because ingredients such as butter, vegetable oil, and/or heavy cream are used in preparation. Instead, choose foods with the words "grilled," "baked," or "light," because these choices are prepared with canola oil instead of lard, vegetable oil, or fatback.

SAMPLE HEALTHY SOUL
FOOD MENU
~
BREAKFAST
Egg white omelet with cheese
Watermelon salad
Fresh berries
~
LUNCH
Hoppin' John (rice and peas)
Collard greens with
smoked turkey necks
~
DINNER
Oven-fried chicken
Ribs, with sauce on the side
Green beans
Baked sweet potato
Buttermilk corn bread
~
DESSERT
Peach crisp
Sweet potato pie

Hoppin' John
The Hoppin' John basics are black-eyed or field peas, rice, onions, bacon, salt, and spices. Try low-fat beef broth instead of bacon and reduce the salt. Eat with collard greens (made without fatback) for a healthy, inexpensive traditional southern U.S. dish.

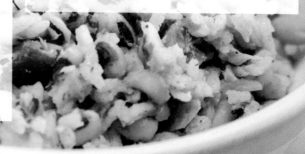

Exercising caution with commercial Chinese food

To maintain your healthy eating goals, there are areas of caution in Chinese feasting, including the fat, sodium, and calorie content of the dishes you select. Deep-fat frying is a common cooking technique for many menu items. Some foods are stir-fried in large amounts of oil and two of the most frequently used flavoring ingredients are monosodium glutamate (MSG) and soy sauce, both of which are high in sodium. However, Chinese cuisine can be enjoyed as part of a sensible diet. Many of the standard dishes consist of noodles or rice built around a variety of vegetables that provide fiber, beta-carotene, vitamin C, and phytonutrients. Tofu or soybean curd provide low-fat, low-cholesterol protein options. Many selections can be steamed, roasted, and simmered, and can form part of your healthier options when on the go.

Pick dishes with these key terms:
Jum—means poached
Kow—means roasted
Shu—means barbecued

Choose spring rolls instead of egg rolls for your appetizer. Both carry similar flavors, but spring rolls will provide fewer calories.

Do not assume that the vegetarian dishes are lower in fat or calories. Many dishes are of the deep-fried varieties. Steamed mixed vegetables will provide vitamins and minerals without the calories. Consider also dishes made with steamed chicken, fish, or shrimp.

The Cantonese variety of Chinese cuisine tends to be lighter because fresh ingredients are part of the tradition. Choose that regional cuisine as much as you can.

Be sensible with sauces. Because sauces can add extra calories, fat, sugar, and sodium to your meal, ask for the sauce on the side so you can decide how much can be added to your meal. Select hoisin, plum, hot mustard, or sweet-and-sour instead of lobster, soy, oyster, and bean sauces. Remember, commercial sauces vary, and some may be higher in calories and sodium than listed, right.

Keep them separate
Asking for steamed veggies? Ask for no added oil and for any sauces to be served on the side.

THE LOWDOWN ON SAUCES (PER TBSP)

Soy
Fat: n/a
Sodium: 1006 mg
Calories: 11
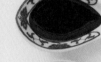

Hoisin
Fat: 1 g
Sodium: 258 mg
Calories: 35

Plum
Fat: n/a
Sodium: 102 mg
Calories: 35
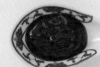

Hot mustard
Fat: n/a
Sodium: 70 mg
Calories: 10

Sweet and sour
Fat: n/a
Sodium: 97 mg
Calories: 22

Black bean
Fat: 1.3 g
Sodium: 500 mg
Calories: 30

Oyster
Fat: n/a
Sodium: 492 mg
Calories: 9

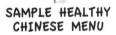

SAMPLE HEALTHY CHINESE MENU
~
APPETIZERS
Spring rolls
Egg drop soup
~
MAINS
Bean curd with sautéed mixed vegetables
Grilled chicken stir-fry with brown rice
~
BEVERAGES
Green tea

Tailor your order
When ordering a chicken stir-fry, ask the restaurant to go light on the oil (for stir-frying), heavy with the veggies, and hold the MSG.

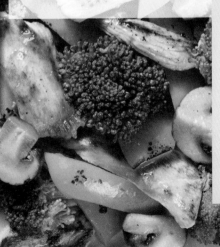

Making Italian meals healthier

Portion sizes are not large and if you choose to eat in the Italian style, the fundamentals of the diet are healthy: high consumption of beans and legumes, fruit and vegetables, grains, and extra virgin olive oil; moderate consumption of wine and dairy products; low consumption of red and processed meat, cream, and pastries.

Superfood your spaghetti dish by opting for vegetarian versions, such as marinara (185 calories per cup) or primavera (223 calories) rather than bolognese (450 calories).

Watch the portion sizes for pasta—$\frac{1}{2}$ to 1 cup per person, especially when it is a side dish to meat, poultry, or fish.

Choose extra virgin olive oil instead of light. This has a stronger flavor, so you can consume less.

Bean-based pasta dishes are both filling and nutritious. Try cannellini in your main dish.

Make your pizza a thin-crust vegetarian at 300 calories, so there's no need to sacrifice this restaurant favorite.

More than a slice of bread
Olive oil imparts flavor and healthy monounsaturated fats; tomatoes provide vitamins C and A and the antioxidant lycopene—great ways to make your bruschetta healthier and delicious.

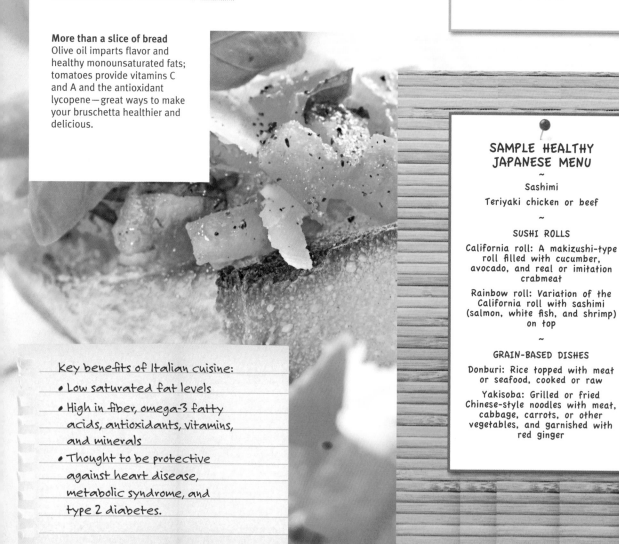

Key benefits of Italian cuisine:
• Low saturated fat levels
• High in fiber, omega-3 fatty acids, antioxidants, vitamins, and minerals
• Thought to be protective against heart disease, metabolic syndrome, and type 2 diabetes.

SAMPLE HEALTHY ITALIAN MENU

~

BREAKFAST
Roll with prosciutto
Fresh fruit salad

~

LUNCH
Bruschetta with tomatoes and olive oil
Shrimp primavera

~

DINNER
Minestrone, Tuscan, or Florentine soup
Vegetarian lasagna

~

DESSERT
Biscotti
Fruit tart

SAMPLE HEALTHY JAPANESE MENU

~

Sashimi
Teriyaki chicken or beef

~

SUSHI ROLLS
California roll: A makizushi-type roll filled with cucumber, avocado, and real or imitation crabmeat

Rainbow roll: Variation of the California roll with sashimi (salmon, white fish, and shrimp) on top

~

GRAIN-BASED DISHES
Donburi: Rice topped with meat or seafood, cooked or raw

Yakisoba: Grilled or fried Chinese-style noodles with meat, cabbage, carrots, or other vegetables, and garnished with red ginger

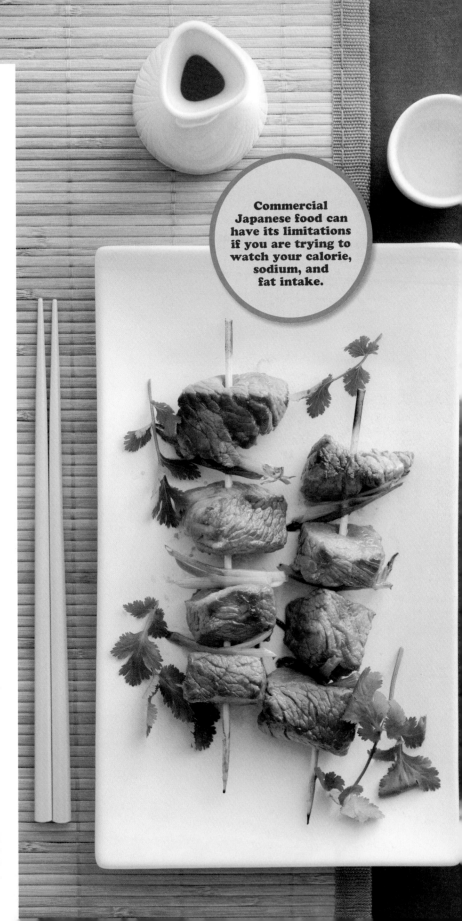

Smart choices with Japanese cuisine

Japanese food is often thought to be healthy since it does not bring fried heavy greasy foods to mind. But the kind of Japanese food that is served outside of Japan can be vastly different than traditional food. With an emphasis on soybeans and rice, it can be a healthy option, if you know what to choose and what to avoid.

Watch the condiments and sauces for sodium—only 1 tablespoon of soy sauce—even the light version—contains almost half the recommended amount of sodium for an entire day.

Pass on rolls and sauces with certain Western ingredients such as cream cheese and mayonnaise.

Limit the "fancy" sushi rolls. The more elaborate rolls such as spider, dynamite, or dragon rolls usually have more than four extra ingredients, as they are often rolled with tempura crumbs or flakes, fish roe, sesame seeds, and drizzled with some kind of sauce. Order two plain, lower-calorie sushi rolls such as salmon, yellowtail, and shrimp rolls instead.

Watch your portions—while rice and noodles are staple ingredients, large helpings of them may not be beneficial. Soba noodles are made with buckwheat, while udon noodles are made out of plain white flour. Soba noodles and brown rice are higher in fiber than udon or white rice.

Steer clear of dishes that include the words "tempura" and "tonkatsu," which means that food is covered with panko (Japanese breadcrumbs) and deep-fried in oil. Choose a dish with steamed, cooked, baked, or grilled ingredients instead.

Consider how it's cooked
Teriyaki is a healthy option due to the cooking process, which involves grilling or broiling.

> Commercial Japanese food can have its limitations if you are trying to watch your calorie, sodium, and fat intake.

113

Maximizing nutrients at a Spanish restaurant

With vegetables, citrus fruit, and seafood at the forefront, Spanish cuisine is an inherently healthy cuisine to turn to for making wholesome dietary choices.

Order two or three tapas for a main meal instead of an entrée. Tapas provide a good opportunity to eat slowly as you chat, so you can be mindful of your appetite as the evening progresses.

Enjoy the many cocidos, or stews with vegetables, popular in Spanish cuisine as a main dish.

Watch the portion size of paella. Often, the waiter will leave the pan with you so you can help yourself. Eat slowly and if you can't resist a second helping, make sure it's smaller than the first, and that it's your last.

If you fancy a meat or tuna pie (empanada) ask the waiter if it can be baked instead of fried.

Sample tomatoes in a variety of ways— drizzled with olive oil as an appetizer, stuffed with rice and vegetables as a main, or as part of a rich stew sauce. A key ingredient in Spanish cuisine, tomatoes are excellent sources of vitamins A and C, and contain the antioxidant lycopene, vitamin E, potassium, and other minerals.

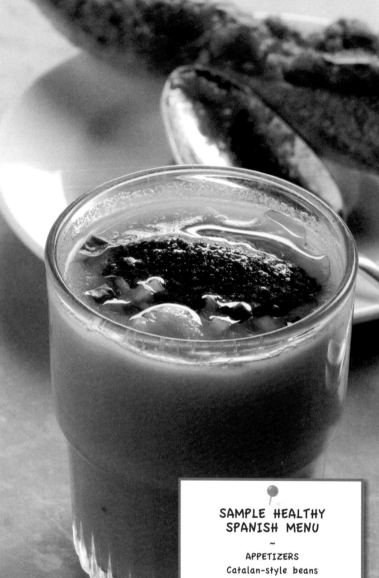

Go easy on the chorizo (Spanish sausage). Just one cup contains 1,120 calories and 132% of your daily allowance of fat.

Ahead of its time
Andalusian gazpacho, here topped with a quenelle of black olives, is a cold tomato-based vegetable soup. The veggies may be finely or coarsely puréed. It's a great low-calorie and nutritious appetizer and, it could be said, a precursor to the popular modern-day veggie smoothies.

SAMPLE HEALTHY
SPANISH MENU
~
APPETIZERS
Catalan-style beans
Gazpacho
~
MAINS
Baked cod and yellow rice
Fabada (bean stew) or fish stew
~
SIDE DISHES
Steamed spinach
Roasted peppers
~
DESSERTS
Almond cookie
Flan

114

SAMPLE HEALTHY MEXICAN MENU

~

APPETIZERS
Salsa with baked corn chips

Caldo de pollo (chicken broth)

~

MAINS
Bean burrito with side salad

Soft corn chicken taco with vegetables

~

SIDE DISHES AND SALSAS
Nopalitos or prickly pear salad

Roasted corn, sweet potato, or other vegetables

~

DESSERTS AND BEVERAGES
Aguas frescas de frutas (fresh fruit drinks)

Rice pudding

Keep an eye on the size

Bean burritos are, on the face of it, a sound option for the health-conscious diner: a flour tortilla filled with mashed beans and rolled, usually with shredded cheese and a sauce included inside the wrap. However, control the portion size and accompaniments to avoid excessive calories.

Enjoying the variety of Mexican food

Mexican food is much more than the commonly known tacos, burritos, enchiladas, and chili. It is varied and colorful, with many healthy staples. Corn, which originated in what is now Mexico, is found in grain as corn tortilla, masa harina (fine cornmeal), and other grain forms, but is also eaten as a vegetable. Black and pinto beans are popular cooked, mashed, or refried.

Many Mexican dishes are "stuffed" foods—tacos, flautas, enchiladas, etc. Be careful to monitor the types and amounts of "stuffings." That's what adds the calories!

Ask about carnes asadas (grilled or roasted meats) and order one with a side of vegetables such as roasted corn.

Like fish tacos? Make sure the fish is not breaded and fried. Sprinkle the tacos with lime instead of dressing.

Enjoy the fruit pastes, but only in small amounts. They are mostly sugar!

Mexican cuisine includes many different types of cheeses, eaten alone, used as toppings, or used in desserts. Weigh up the calorie, fat, and calcium content when making your menu choices.

Panela Usually eaten fresh as a snack or over cold dishes. 1 oz = 80 calories, 4 g saturated fat, 15% calcium.

Queso blanco A crumbly cheese used as a topping, or creamy when heated. Avoid it in frying. 1 oz = 90 calories; 4 g saturated fat, 20% calcium.

Queso fresco A common crumbly Mexican cheese used as a topping and to stuff quesadillas and chilies. 1 oz = 87 calories, 4 g saturated fat, 16% calcium.

Crema Like a thick heavy or sour cream, used in sauces or toppings. 1 oz = 60 calories, 3.5 g saturated fat, 2% calcium.

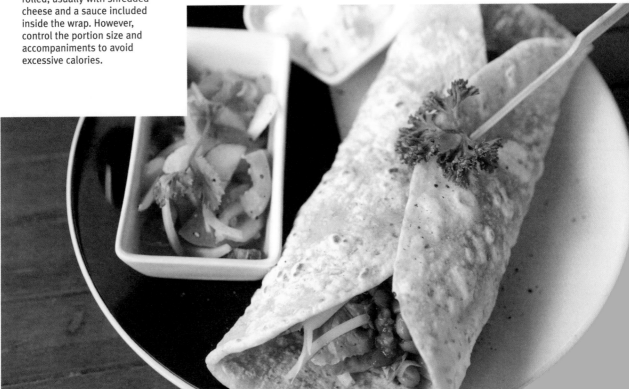

Healthy choices at parties

Party time should be when you get to savor delicious foods while supporting, not sabotaging, your eating goals. Then you can savor the fun, too.

For many people, party times can be a source of stress and worry, since they may be tempted to deviate from their healthy eating goals. The key to enjoying the celebration and the food is to know what type of event you are hosting or attending, the types of foods and beverages that are likely to be there, and to develop a strategy for enjoying the event.

Be mindful of requirements

If hosting, ask your guests to let you know in advance of any special dietary requirements. Make sure your menu suits all your guests, tailor it to do so, or provide suitable alternatives. For example, if you have nuts as an appetizer (and a person with nut allergies attending), provide popcorn or another item, too. Also keep "high allergy" foods away from commonly selected items to avoid cross-contamination.

If you're planning to attend a party, ask the host in advance what dishes will be served. If they are not likely to have low-fat and healthy options, or options that cater to your special dietary requirements, offer to bring some to help out. Once there, check out all the tasty treats on offer before eating or drinking anything. Plan on a few items from the major categories—appetizers, main dishes, side dishes, sweets, and beverages. Have an idea of portions and maximum limits before digging in.

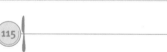

115

Avoid mindless drinking and eating

At the party, limit what you eat by holding a glass of sparkling water with one hand and a celery stick with the other hand. Your hands will be too full to let you mindlessly eat other higher-calorie foods.

116

Create a theme with the decor

If you want to create a theme, do it through the decorations around the environment rather than the food. For example, a New Year's party with a blue-and-silver color scheme could have balloons and confetti in blue and silver around small cupcakes instead of cupcakes covered with dark-blue frosting. Or you could serve ladyfingers, angel cake, or sponge topped with blueberries.

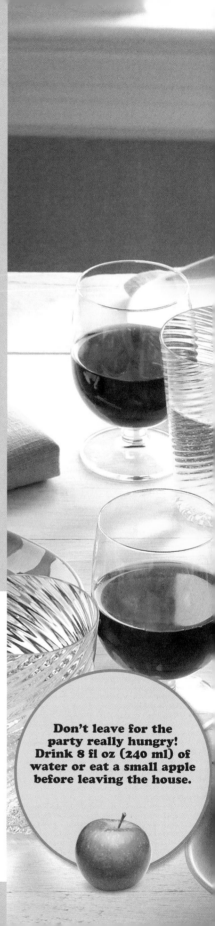

Don't leave for the party really hungry! Drink 8 fl oz (240 ml) of water or eat a small apple before leaving the house.

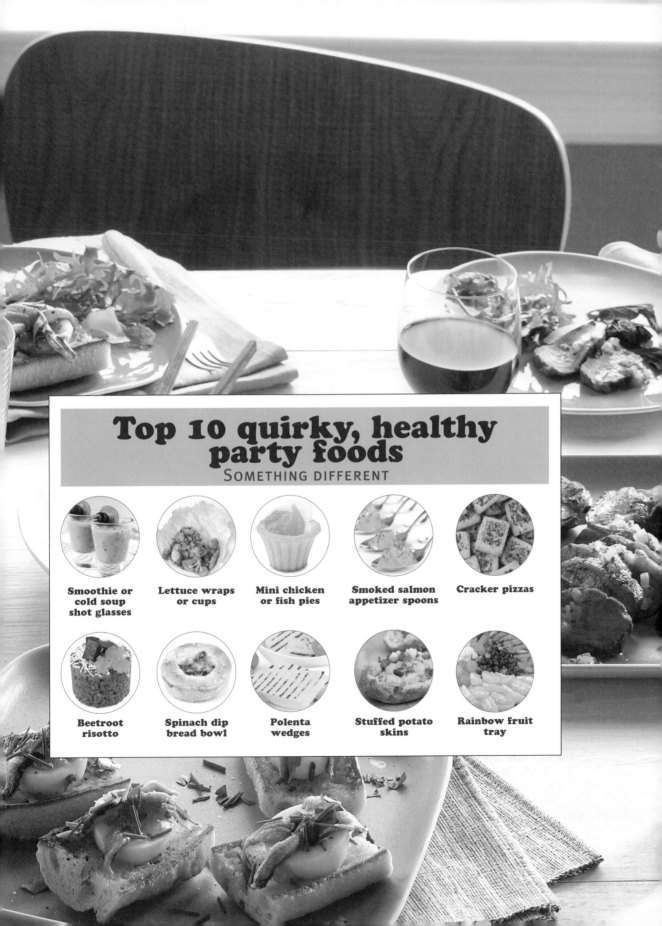

Top 10 quirky, healthy party foods

SOMETHING DIFFERENT

Smoothie or cold soup shot glasses

Lettuce wraps or cups

Mini chicken or fish pies

Smoked salmon appetizer spoons

Cracker pizzas

Beetroot risotto

Spinach dip bread bowl

Polenta wedges

Stuffed potato skins

Rainbow fruit tray

Start the party right—appetizers

Many appetizers are laden with cheese or sauces or fried to a crisp. With a few wise choices, however, appetizers can remain delicious but also be healthy.

Appetizers are a great idea, but unfortunately many are made up of heavy dips or cheese-stuffed items that contain as many—if not more—calories than the meal itself. The good news is that by focusing on unique uses of healthy foods such as fruits, vegetables, and low-calorie proteins instead, you can quickly turn the appetizer into a guilt-free, full-flavor home run.

Serve "complicated" finger foods

Nuts in their shells, such as pistachios and peanuts, require work to eat and will naturally help you eat less. Other foods that take a little work are mollusks (clams, oysters, and mussels), shell-on shrimp, or edamame.

Don't scrimp on the salsa!

Salsa is one condiment that you can always feel good about serving because it's full of flavor and vegetables and low in calories—only 30 per tablespoon. Serve it with fresh vegetable slices, low-calorie crackers, or baked chips. Salsa is also versatile because you can use it as a dip—or for a topping on finger sandwiches or other foods. It's an easy way to enhance an appetizer with minimal work.

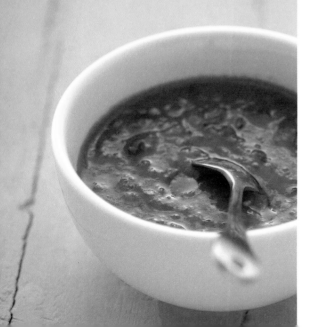

When choosing appetizers at a party, rather than putting a little of everything on your plate, look through the whole selection first, and then decide on two to three items to enjoy.

Sarah-Jane Bedwell, author of *Schedule Me Skinny*

Prime position

The placement of your appetizers can be a strategy to help you and your guests make the best choices. Put fruits and vegetables at the front and center positions in the serving area and set higher-calorie appetizers farther away. Research has shown that the farther you have to walk for food, the less likely you are to choose it.

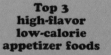

Top 3 high-flavor low-calorie appetizer foods
1 Roasted vegetables
2 Raw fruit
3 Grilled shrimp skewers

End the party right—sweets

Healthy eating at a party does not mean you should skip the sweets or desserts table. It means finding a way to indulge without compromising your health goals.

One strategy for enjoying sweets but avoiding excess is to fill up on healthy snacks and foods before walking to the dessert table so you are not as tempted to overeat desserts and sweets. However, you can indulge sensibly with smaller portions or healthier versions of your favorite desserts and still have fun alongside everyone else at the party.

In most recipes, you can decrease the amount of sugar by up to one third or fat by up to a half and still have a delicious treat.

 120

Control your ingredients

Think carefully before choosing store-bought sweet rolls, cookies, pies, cakes, and cream-filled desserts. These foods are usually high in sugar and unhealthy fats, such as trans or saturated fats. Making your own desserts means you can lower the amount of added sugar or fats.

 122

Healthy party desserts

Make your frosting with Neufchâtel cheese and a small amount of powdered sugar instead of a large amount of cream cheese or butter and sugar.

Instead of frosting a chocolate cake, place a doily over the cake, sprinkle powdered sugar, and then remove the doily to reveal an attractive pattern.

Serve small biscottis instead of cakes or cookies.

Make pies with a lattice top with large open spaces to have less pie crust and fewer calories.

Use whisky cups to replace regular cups for ice cream and provide nut toppings instead of syrups.

121

Chocolate-covered strawberries

Chocolate may reduce the risk of heart disease, and dark chocolate may have better health benefits than milk chocolate. Combine with fruit for added health benefits, and taste.

Ingredients
- 20 strawberries
- 6 oz (170 g) dark chocolate, chopped

Directions

1. Melt the chocolate in a glass dish in the microwave, then let it cool slightly and thicken.

2. Hold each strawberry by the stem and dip then twist the bottom half in the melted chocolate.

52 calories and 2.6 g fat per strawberry

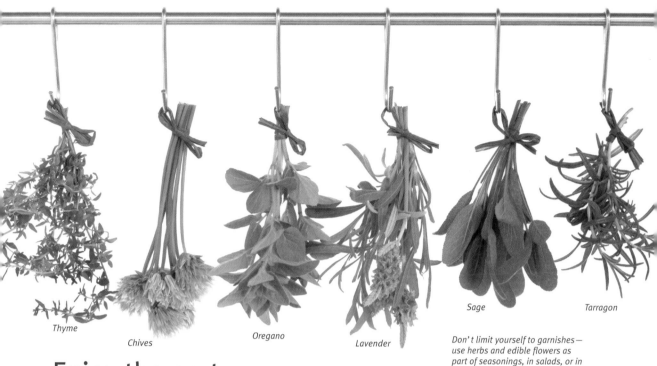

Thyme

Chives

Oregano

Lavender

Sage

Tarragon

Don't limit yourself to garnishes—
use herbs and edible flowers as
part of seasonings, in salads, or in
vinegars for a culinary treat.

Enjoy the party—
right! Main dishes

Whether you are providing, bringing, or just eating, focus
on reducing the fat and calories in main dishes.

With a little effort and forethought, it's nearly always possible to reduce the
calories in a dish. However, choosing low-calorie in the first place could make
things easier. So why not try soups or stews, for example, and make them broth-
based rather than cream-based? Many recipes allow you take advantage of each
season's bountiful produce and spices, e.g. vegetable noodle soup in the spring
or pumpkin soup in the fall. Comforting, vegetable-filled casseroles can be a great
winter warmer for large gatherings, with brown rice and whole-grain bread to
increase fiber intake. Whole-grain vegetarian pizzas are ideal for sharing, and there
are many healthy salads that add flavor, texture, and nutrients as a side dish or
on their own.

124

Rely on herbs

Fresh herbs are a wonderful addition to
any cold dish because they add vibrant
flavor and antioxidants. Because heat
tends to amplify flavors, cold dishes
really benefit from the extra flavor-boost
herbs provide.

125

Pasta appeal

Often found at parties, a filling, healthy
pasta salad can easily be created by
using a handful of vegetables and a few
splashes of dressing. It can be a
surprisingly filling dish: if the salad
contains high-fiber grains and beans,
such as quinoa, barley, wheatberries,
bulgur wheat, black beans, or kidney
beans in place of pasta, it will fill you up
on less quantity and calories. These
substitutions are great options for people
who need to control their blood sugar or
just want to eat low-glycemic-index foods.

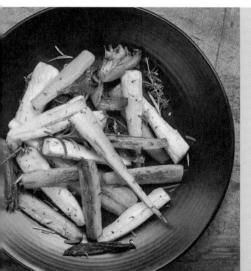

123

Roast veggies for a
colorful, healthy dish

For a tasty side dish, toss chopped
parsnips, carrots, and Brussels
sprouts evenly in olive oil and herbs
and roast or grill. Roasting vegetables
like bell peppers, jalapeños, carrots,
parsnips, and eggplant will bring out
complex, sweet flavors. Pay attention
to presentation by considering colors,
herb toppings, and serving dishes.

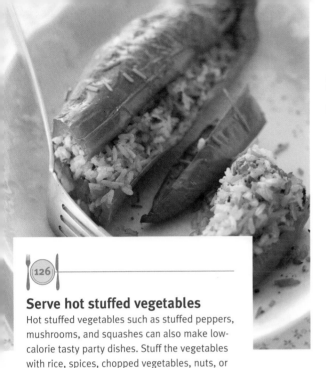

128
Cooking with cheese

Choose reduced-fat or low-fat cheeses such as skim milk mozzarella, string cheese, or Jarlsberg light for casseroles. When trying reduced-fat forms of cheeses such as Cheddar, Monterey Jack, Brie, Swiss, Colby, Muenster, and American in cooking, avoid very high temperatures, which may make them—and your dish—rubbery.

129
Healthy substitutions

Instead of...	Try this...
Mayonnaise	Low-fat Greek yogurt
Creamy dressings	Red wine vinegar
Butter	Small amounts of olive oil
Salt, to boost flavor	Fresh herbs

126
Serve hot stuffed vegetables

Hot stuffed vegetables such as stuffed peppers, mushrooms, and squashes can also make low-calorie tasty party dishes. Stuff the vegetables with rice, spices, chopped vegetables, nuts, or lean meats. Use lean ground turkey or beef instead of higher-fat beef to reduce the fat intake. To add a nutty flavor and boost the nutrition even further, substitute white rice with brown rice or whole-grain breadcrumbs.

127

serves 10

Wholesome pasta salad

This pasta salad maximizes the use of vegetables and, with plenty of green and red, makes for an attractive dish on your party table.

Ingredients
- 1½ cups dry whole-grain, short-cut pasta (gemelli, macaroni, or rotini)
- 2 tablespoons extra virgin olive oil
- 4 tablespoons red wine vinegar
- 3 tablespoons minced fresh parsley
- Zest of one lemon
- 1 cup chopped cherry tomatoes
- 3 cups fresh spinach
- 1 zucchini, diced
- 1 red bell pepper, diced
- 1 cup small-cut broccoli florets
- 3 tablespoons diced scallions

Per ½ cup serving: 105 calories, 3.2 g fat, 0.4 g saturated fat, 0 g trans fat, 0 mg cholesterol, 16 g carbohydrate, 3.3 g fiber, 1.2 g sugar, 4 g protein

Directions

1. Cook pasta according to the directions on the box.

2. In a small bowl, whisk together the oil, vinegar, herbs, and lemon zest.

3. Drain the pasta, and then put it into a large serving bowl. Add the spinach immediately and toss into the pasta until slightly wilted.

4. Add the remainder of the vegetables, scallions, and dressing, and toss to fully coat.

5. Refrigerate for at least two hours until chilled. Serve cold.

A filling, healthy pasta salad can be created easily by using a handful of vegetables and a few splashes of dressing.

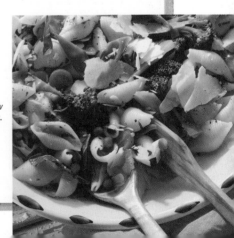

Healthy drinking practices

Sugar-sweetened or alcohol-containing beverages can contribute a surprising number of calories to your diet at party time. Drink smart, and you can still enjoy the good times.

Keep your punch healthy and cold by freezing fruit in diet ginger ale or sparkling water in a mold and inverting into your punch prior to serving.

Whether it is soda, tea, eggnog, beer, wine, or hard liquor, there are three main things you need to watch out for:
• Alcohol
• Sugar
• Calories
There are several strategies you can use to enjoy the party while staying healthy and happy.

Limiting alcohol

If you plan on treating yourself to a glass of alcohol, start with a calorie-free, non-alcoholic beverage such as sparkling water with lime to satisfy your thirst and save you some calories before you have your alcoholic drink. You may have a glass of light beer, wine, bourbon, rum, vodka, gin, or a mixed drink, but red wine is a slightly better choice: in moderate amounts it provides antioxidants and offers heart-healthy benefits.

To avoid drinking too much, you can dilute alcoholic drinks with water or juice. Ask for a spritzer such as wine with club soda or diet ginger ale. You may ask for an addition of antioxidant-high cranberry juice or vitamin C-high lime juice and create your own wine spritzer. Know your limit and drink in moderation—approximately one serving of an alcoholic beverage per hour is the general rate of consumption for adequate metabolism. Having too much alcohol may put you at risk of intoxication and dangerous driving. A general recommendation is a maximum of one drink per day for women and two drinks per day for men.

Beware the empty calories

Having too many sugary drinks will result in taking in lots of empty calories with little or no nutritional value. This becomes especially easy because you may be "drinking mindlessly." That is, because you are involved in talking or other activities you are not aware of how much you are drinking. Prior to

What else can you drink?

If you want to avoid alcohol altogether, there are some tasty and refreshing alternatives you can turn to:
• Plain water, with a slice lemon or lime for a fresh taste
• Sparkling or tonic water with a splash of 100% fruit juice
• 100% fruit juice (a small amount)
• Unsweetened iced tea or sweetened with calorie-free sweeteners
• Diet soda

attending the party, set yourself a limit of sugar-sweetened drinks or alcoholic drinks and be aware of how many calories each contains.

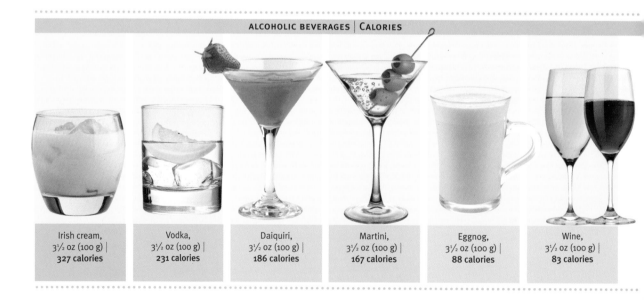

ALCOHOLIC BEVERAGES | CALORIES

Irish cream, 3½ oz (100 g)	**327 calories**
Vodka, 3½ oz (100 g)	**231 calories**
Daiquiri, 3½ oz (100 g)	**186 calories**
Martini, 3½ oz (100 g)	**167 calories**
Eggnog, 3½ oz (100 g)	**88 calories**
Wine, 3½ oz (100 g)	**83 calories**

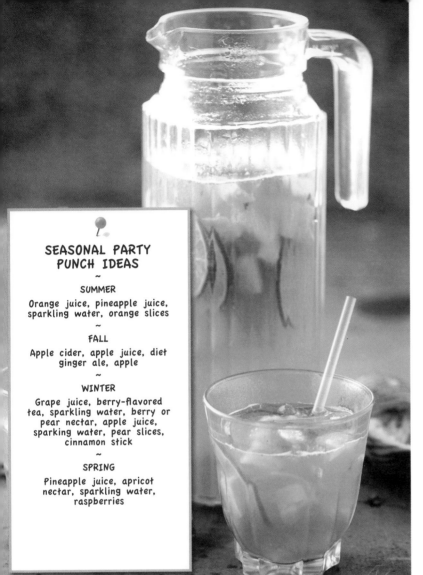

SEASONAL PARTY PUNCH IDEAS

~

SUMMER
Orange juice, pineapple juice, sparkling water, orange slices

~

FALL
Apple cider, apple juice, diet ginger ale, apple

~

WINTER
Grape juice, berry-flavored tea, sparkling water, berry or pear nectar, apple juice, sparking water, pear slices, cinnamon stick

~

SPRING
Pineapple juice, apricot nectar, sparkling water, raspberries

131

Explore healthy hot drink options

On some occasions such as holiday parties in the winter, hot drinks keep you warm and healthy. As a host, you may offer some flavored teas. Tea contains antioxidants and other compounds and may prevent against cancer, heart disease, and other diseases. Choose unsweetened brewed tea over sweetened to avoid extra calorie intake from sugar. Another option is herbal teas such as ginger, jasmine, and mint. Herbal teas are caffeine-free or lower-caffeine beverages made from herbs, flowers, roots, bark, and seeds steeped in hot water. Some may have anti-inflammatory properties.

132

Drink in moderation

Drink water between alcoholic beverages to dilute the effects of alcohol. Sip alcoholic beverages slowly and leave a gap between glasses.

NON-ALCOHOLIC BEVERAGES | CALORIES

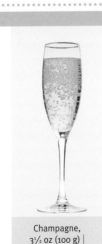

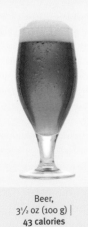

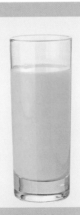

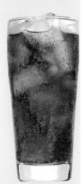

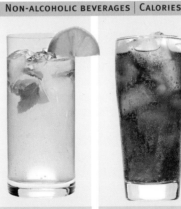

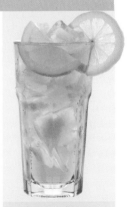

| Champagne, 3½ oz (100 g) \| **76 calories** | Beer, 3½ oz (100 g) \| **43 calories** | Orange juice, 8 fl oz (230 ml) \| **111 calories** | Lemonade, 8 fl oz (230 ml) \| **99 calories** | Cola, 8 fl oz (230 ml) \| **92 calories** | Unsweetened iced tea, 8 fl oz (230 ml) \| **92 calories** |

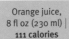

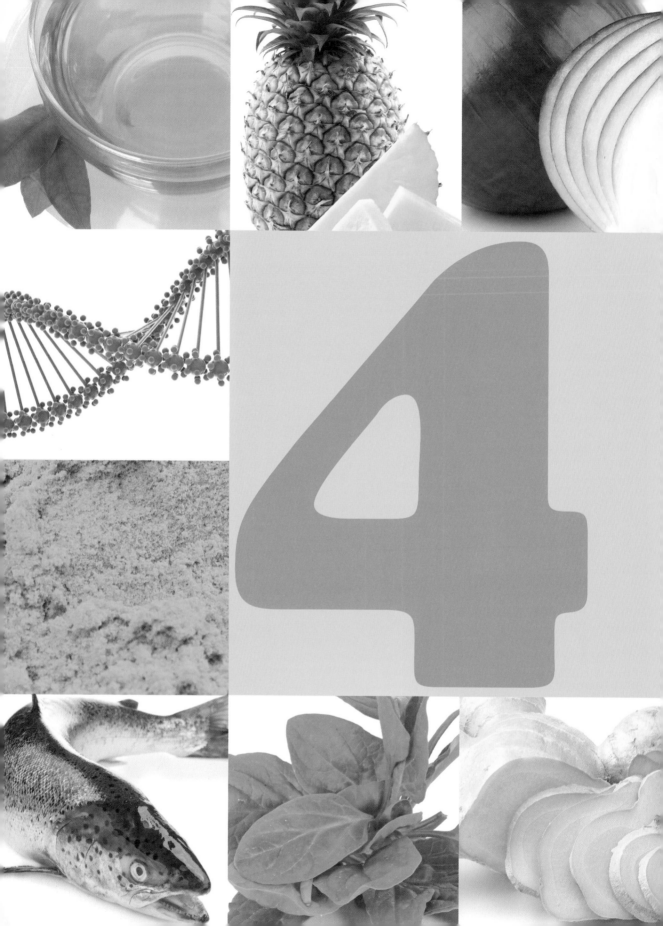

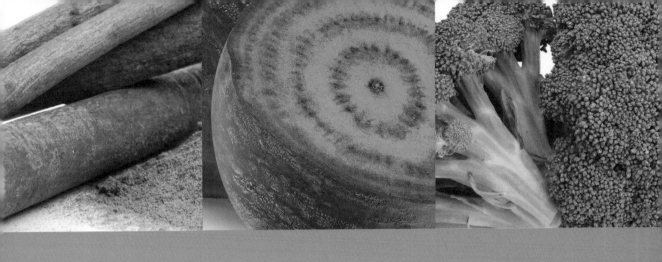

Diets and eating plans

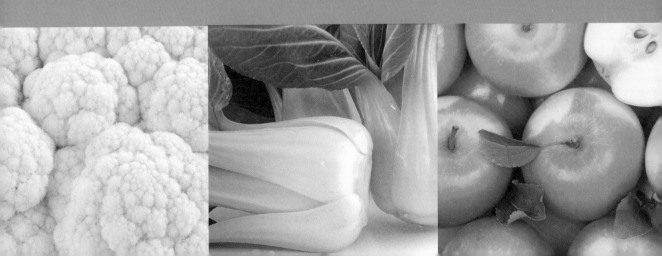

Popular diets and plans

Okay, you've heard it before. Diets don't work. But you want to try that "hot" new diet. Should you? Find out if it may work for you, and how to do it safely, if at all.

Do this...

✓ Spend your money on a trained professional, such as a registered or licensed dietitian/nutritionist, who can personalize a plan based on your needs.

...Not this

✗ Spend your money on a million-dollar bestseller that will collect dust on your shelf.

You may have modified how you eat or bought a weight-loss book in order to lose weight. But think about it: If you spent money on a diet book, did you lose anything permanently other than the money?

Most diets work in the short term because they encourage you to lower your total calorie intake. They do this through a variety of different techniques—see the chart, right.

Keep in mind that because a diet is popular, that does not necessarily mean it is safe or is based on studies of its effectiveness. The best diet for you is the one that was specifically designed for you, and considers your likes and dislikes, your financial limits, your lifestyle and weight, and your health goals. A registered or licensed dietitian/nutritionist can help you with this.

No matter the diet and its claims, what you should look for in any diet is its EAT factor:

Ease of incorporation given your eating behaviors, likes, current finances, and need for long-term use.

Application to your lifestyle and situation; "family friendliness."

Truthfulness of claims—does the science really support that it is safe and is effective?

(133)

Start small and specific
Start by setting one small goal every two weeks, such as replacing lunchtime French fries with a side salad on Mondays, Wednesdays, and Fridays.

(134)

Don't believe the hype
What is the diet claim? Lose weight fast? Cleanse you? Build muscle without exercise? How much does it cost? You know it's not true. Save your money and follow a free plan instead of buying in to unproven marketing claims.

(135)

Five diet myths
An informed dieter is a smarter—and therefore more successful—dieter. Make sure you separate fact from fiction. Here are some popular misconceptions about dieting:

1 Skip meals to lose weight.

2 Diet foods are best for weight loss.

3 Starches are fattening.

4 Low-fat or fat-free foods are lower in calories.

5 You cannot eat out when trying to lose weight.

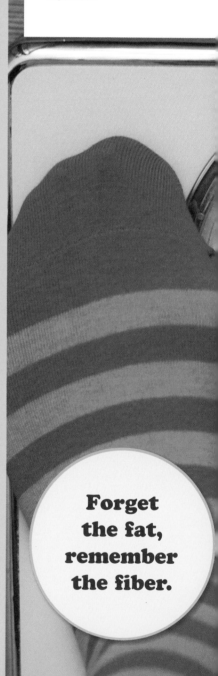

Forget the fat, remember the fiber.

Technique	Key attributes and practices	Example diets
Behavior change	Healthy eating, physical activity, and behavior changes; i.e. using smaller plates, cue identification, regular exercise	➤ French women's diet ➤ Intuitive eating ➤ Mindful eating
Consumption of foods in specific combinations or preparation	Eating or not eating specific foods together, or only prepared in specific ways	➤ Fit for life ➤ Raw food diet (pages 100–101)
Consumption of specific foods at set times	Eating or not eating specific foods at specific times	➤ 3-hour diet
Consumption of foods based on typing or classification of population groups	Encouraging you to classify yourself according to groups such as blood type	➤ Eat right for your type
Focus on consumption of one or a few specific foods	Eating a specific food for its "special qualities"	➤ Grapefruit diet ➤ Cabbage soup diet ➤ Vegan diet (pages 102–103) ➤ Paleo diet (pages 106–107)
Personalized guidance based on lifestyle, health, and genetic predispositions (pages 94–95)	Personalizing your plan based on your health goals, lifestyle, preferences, and disease risk	➤ Fat is not your fate ➤ Forever young
Restriction of proteins, fats, or carbohydrates	Limiting your intake of one or two of the macronutrients	➤ New Atkins diet ➤ Dukan diet ➤ South Beach diet
Purchase and consumption of meal replacements	Using commercial beverages, snacks, and/or meal replacements	➤ Jenny Craig ➤ Weight Watchers ➤ Slimfast ➤ Nutrisystem
Total or partial avoidance of foods (pages 98–99)	Encouraging you to fast	➤ Daniel fast ➤ Juice fast diet ➤ Intermittent 5:2 diet
Food groups and exchanges	Selecting foods from categories or groups to create menus or snacks within established limits	➤ Volumetrics ➤ DASH diet (pages 104–105)
Techniques that "remove toxins or cleanse" (pages 96–97)	Encouraging you to "detox" by fasting or promoting foods that supposedly eliminate toxins	➤ Green smoothie detox diet ➤ Super cleanse

Working with a registered dietitian/nutritionist

Whether you want to lose weight, eat to manage your diabetes, or just learn some healthy food tips to implement in family meals, consider working with a nutrition professional.

Often, you may think you are making the best selections and be unaware of strategies you can use to improve your choices. In much the same way you would see a physician when you are ill, or a dentist for prophylactic care or treatment, you should consider working with a qualified nutritionist such as a registered dietitian/nutritionist who can help you establish and succeed with your food and nutrition goals. Working with a nutrition professional will help you identify your needs and set a course of action that fits your lifestyle and goals.

What should you look for when seeking a qualified professional?

Ask the practitioner if he or she has a degree in nutrition and dietetics. Ask where he or she studied—was it an accredited program? Ask the potential consultant if he or she took courses such as chemistry, anatomy and physiology, food science and food safety, nutrition science, dietetics, and medical nutrition therapy. Also, did the practitioner have clinical or internship experience? Does the practitioner belong to a professional organization such as the Academy of Nutrition and Dietetics? Does the professional take regular continuing education courses to stay up to date? What is the practitioner's area of practice? Is it related your counseling needs?

One easy way to find a registered dietitian/nutritionist is to find out the name of the professional organization, such as the Academy of Nutrition and Dietetics (United States), Dietitians of Canada, etc. They can provide you with names of local practitioners who are consultants.

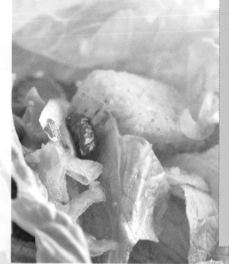

Five questions to ask a potential consultant to determine if the nutritionist is qualified to counsel you

1 How long was your program of study?

2 Did you do an accredited internship or supervised practice program?

3 Are you registered with the Commission on Dietetic Registration?

4 Are you licensed?

5 What is your practice specialty area?

If you answer "yes" to any of the questions below, you might find it beneficial to work with a dietitian/nutritionist. Do you find it hard to:

• Analyze different diets and diet claims for hype and truth?

• Figure out how to create a weight-loss diet that works for you?

• Figure out what to look for on a food's nutrition label?

• Make sense of the items listed on a food's Ingredients List?

• Plan meals that are quick, healthy, and delicious?

• Plan meals that fit your goals but also please other family members?

• Buy foods that help you and your family prevent disease?

• Buy the foods you need for your special diet?

• Buy a range of foods but stay within a budget?

• Make healthy snacks or meals to eat on the move?

• Eat healthily when eating out?

Going for a consultation?
Be prepared to provide information about your health status, medications, diets you have tried in the past, and the current or expected diet. Keep track of what you generally eat (see below) and write questions you want to ask.

A typical session
A health professional will likely help you identify your eating patterns, behaviors, and goals. The assessment may include the use of 24-hour recalls—where you identify everything you ate over the past 24 hours or previous day, including nutrition information—and helping you to identify goal-setting health behaviors, and discussing possible barriers and supports in relation to achieving those goals.

See a qualified professional
Make sure you ask the potential consultant questions. In some areas, the term "nutritionist" can only be used by a trained, qualified professional, but in other places the term can be used by anyone! The term "registered dietitian" is usually more closely regulated for use by trained health professionals. But do not take anything for granted—ask about the consultant's credentials and training.

Check these out
U.S. Academy of Nutrition and Dietetics: www.eatright.org
Provides nutrition information and videos on a variety of topics and contact details of possible consultants.

The Bristish Dietetic Association: www.bda.uk.com
Freelance Dietitians: www.freelancedietitians.org
Find a dietitian in the U.K.

Dietitians in Canada: www.dietitians.ca
Find a dietitian in Canada.

Be honest in your diet record to give the nutritionist a true picture of your eating habits. Only then will he or she be able to help you.

Recording your eating habits
To make the most of your time with a registered dietitian, keep a diet record. For three to five days prior to the visit (include at least one weekend day) write down everything you eat, how much, where you got it from (was it made at home or bought in a restaurant?). Try to include level of hunger (1 = not hungry to 4 = extremely hungry) and emotional state such as bored, happy, sad, angry. Keeping a diet record that is based on how you actually eat will allow a dietitian to make an accurate assessment. Changing your eating habits or skipping writing down some items you eat will hinder your chances of working together successfully. A sample diet record might look like this:

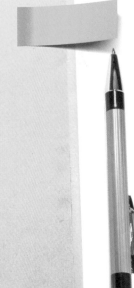

MEAL OR SNACK? 1pm Snack

FOOD OR DISH
• Spanish omelet
• 16 oz orange juice

INGREDIENTS
1 egg, ½ medium sliced fried potato, ¼ cup onion

LOCATION
Bought and ate at café

HUNGER LEVEL
2 A bit hungry, very thirsty

EMOTION
Upset over work issue

Nutrigenomics: What's in it for you?

Based on knowledge of your specific genetic risks, a dietitian/nutritionist can personalize your plan and tailor your food choices to meet your individual needs. No more one-size-fits-all diet plans.

The best weight-loss diet is the one that is planned especially for you!

The future is bright in that it will be possible to design health care especially for you. In five to ten years, with valid and reliable genetic testing and advancing research on functional food ingredients (foods or ingredients made for a specific purpose) to change gene expression (such as decreasing your risk for diabetes), personalized nutrition will be the new diet. What will

it look like? Today, we can make general recommendations for specific diet types depending on family history and disease risk (see below). However, in the future, people will have a gene map and know what diseases their genes predict in 10, 20, 30, or 40-plus years and what foods can affect the expression of those genes by turning them on or off to reduce risk.

This will require a lot of research to identify the disease risk genes (this is already happening), identify the food ingredients that can modify the expression of those genes (this will take longer), and then determine the right time to eat those foods, as there are critical periods for changing gene expression. Here is an example of a critical period: Preliminary evidence indicates that foods containing soy eaten during puberty may reduce the risk of breast cancer in later life but have no positive effect if started after menopause. Another example may be that some people will lose weight on a higher-carbohydrate low-protein diet, while others may respond better to a low-carbohydrate high-protein diet.

> " The future is fast approaching and the diets of that future will be informed by genetic information about each patient. "

Catherine Christie, Associate Dean and Professor, University of North Florida

Examples of personalized eating strategies

You can't change your parents, but you can change your behaviors

You cannot alter your genetic predisposition—the likelihood of getting a disease based on your genetic makeup, or what you inherited from your ancestors (such as potential for type 2 diabetes)—but you can decrease the potential of getting that disease by avoiding related risk factors.

Kidney disease risk
If kidney disease runs in your family, keeping blood pressure under control is critical. Avoid high-sodium and processed foods as much as possible and keep weight under control.

Heart disease risk
If heart disease runs in your family, avoid smoking or other tobacco products. Eating a heart-healthy calorie-balanced diet with predominantly monounsaturated and polyunsaturated fat sources makes sense. Limit saturated fat and avoid becoming overweight. Learn to like foods and their natural flavor—without added salt—and monitor blood pressure regularly. Learn to handle stress and stay physically active most days of the week.

Have a session in a Bod Pod

Have a qualified professional measure your body composition in a Bod Pod, if you have access. You sit inside the large egg-shaped piece of equipment for a few seconds and a qualified health professional will then interpret the results. It's an accurate and efficient way to assess your body composition—how much fat and muscle you have and your resting metabolic rate.

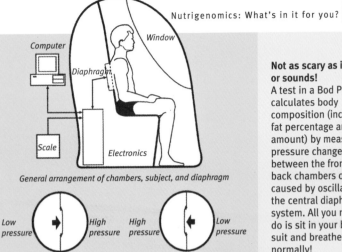

General arrangement of chambers, subject, and diaphragm

Moving diaphragm produces complementary pressure changes in the chambers

Not as scary as it looks, or sounds!
A test in a Bod Pod calculates body composition (including fat percentage and amount) by measuring pressure changes between the front and back chambers of the Pod caused by oscillations of the central diaphragm system. All you need to do is sit in your bathing suit and breathe normally!

Access and ethics

Genetic testing is currently available in some parts of the world over the counter and direct to consumers without medical professional interpretation or involvement. This has raised red flags because of lab-testing inconsistencies and the recommendations of supplements for sale by the same companies who provide the test. Privacy concerns have also been raised in that employers or insurance companies might request predictive genetic information and deny employment or coverage based on future risk.

In the meantime, as we wait for these ethical and other issues to be solved, diets should be personalized as much as possible using what we currently know about family history and disease risk.

Accuracy in predicting what is best for each patient based on his or her genes will increase drastically. Skill in helping patients to change their eating and exercise behaviors will depend on our understanding of the behavior-change process and the development and provision of the ideal foods and ingredients for each genotype.

Breast cancer risk

If breast cancer runs in your family, consider working to prevent excess weight gain with age. Limit alcohol intake and tobacco use and focus on a diet high in vegetables, fruits, poultry, fish, and low-fat dairy products. If skin cancer runs in your family, keep skin protected and always use sunscreen. For other cancers, follow the same rules as for breast cancer until more specific recommendations emerge from the research.

Diabetes risk

If diabetes runs in your family, keeping extra weight off in childhood, early adulthood, and middle adulthood is a smart strategy. Emphasizing aerobic exercise for calorie burning and restricting high-calorie foods and beverages makes sense. Limiting non-nutrient-dense foods such as desserts, sweetened beverages, and chips and snack foods may also be prudent. It would also be important to know precisely how many calories you burn in a day so intake can be adjusted. This can be done using a Bod Pod (see above) or underwater weighing.

 Do this...

✓ Talk with your family members about their health conditions and discuss them with your physician and dietitian.

 ...Not this

✗ Spend your money on a mail-order "saliva test" that claims to see if you are at risk for diseases and health conditions. The method has not yet been fully demonstrated to be effective or standardized for valid results.

Detox diets

Detox diets are very short-term options that may have some benefits, but only if done in the right way, if you are healthy, and if you can manage them.

It is important to consult your doctor before starting a detox diet, to make sure that certain foods are not harmful to you.

The need for detoxification diets comes from the idea that the tissues of your body store up pollutants and toxins from the environment, poor diets, and medications. By fasting for a set period of time from the typical Western diet, and choosing mostly plant-based foods, it is thought that the body's natural detoxification system can be accelerated or enhanced.

Your body, however, is equipped to naturally detoxify every day. The liver's main function is to filter the blood (to remove waste), detoxify chemicals, and break down drugs. This is a crucial role that supports overall health. In extreme cases, when the liver is not healthy or able to detoxify properly, by-products of metabolism, alcohol, or drugs can build up in the blood, causing illness and perhaps even leading to death.

Helping your liver to help itself

An overall healthy diet is the key to keeping your liver running on all cylinders. A wide variety and ample intake of fruits and vegetables is the first and most important component of a detoxification diet. Specifically, produce that contains sulfur compounds—such as onions, garlic, broccoli, cabbage, kale, cauliflower, and Brussels sprouts—is particularly well equipped to provide nutrients to power the liver. These foods should be enjoyed daily in both raw and cooked forms.

Spices like turmeric and cinnamon have also been found to support the liver's function and should be used for flavoring instead of salt or added fat. Fruits like apples and pineapples contain important enzymes and nutrients that aid in breaking down food and eliminating waste.

Steering clear

There are a few things that should be avoided while following a detox diet. Having to metabolize alcohol and foods high in fat such as fried foods diverts the liver from performing its other important functions. It is also recommended to avoid caffeine and instead drink water and hot decaffeinated green tea.

EVERYDAY TIPS

1 Eat a fruit or vegetable at every meal. This will help support your body's natural detoxification system.

2 Foods that contain certain phytonutrients support the liver's process for detoxifying at the cellular level.

3 Keep caffeinated beverages to one a day or less and drink lots of water and green tea instead.

4 Drink alcohol only on occasion (one to two times a week or less) to support a healthy liver.

5 Prefer spices and herbs daily over salt and extra fat.

Pros	Cons
Mentally, following a "detox" diet plan for a short period of time can help to jump-start health and better decision-making, through eating more fruit and vegetables.	Although the science is not strong, preliminary research suggests that detox diets are not a good way to lose weight and keep it off.
Although it may seem contradictory, "detoxing" is something that can be achieved every day by eating, not avoiding, healthy foods.	There are a host of supplements and food replacements sold as part of a "detox" regimen that are best avoided. Most are laxatives, and many could be unsafe or harmful.
Following a detox plan can heighten your awareness of the keys to feeling great and having a healthy liver for life.	Strict plans carried out over long periods of time or that rely on supplements are generally considered unsafe, and there's no proof that they offer benefits.

145   DETOX PLAN

sample menu

~

BREAKFAST

Whole-food smoothie made of fresh orange, apple, kale, carrots, ginger, and turmeric

Hot green tea

~

LUNCH

Cooked quinoa or brown rice with chopped tomatoes, lettuce, avocado, and broccoli

~

SNACK

Fresh berries sprinkled with cinnamon

~

DINNER

Brussels sprouts roasted with garlic
Miso soup

Top 9 foods
TO SUPPORT DETOXIFICATION

Cauliflower   **Onions**   **Apples**

Green tea   **Cinnamon**   **Beets**

Turmeric   **Fresh ginger**   **Pineapple**

Detox smoothie

146

serves 1

Try this smoothie as an easy way to get several of the top detox foods in your diet daily.

Ingredients

½ cup carrot juice

½ cup water

1 cup fresh kale

1 medium apple, cut into chunks

¼ cup fresh or frozen pineapple chunks

1-inch (2.5-cm) piece of fresh ginger root

1 tablespoon turmeric

Directions

Put all ingredients in a blender and process until smooth. Add more water if necessary to achieve your preferred consistency.

176 calories, 2 g total fat, 0 g saturated fat, 0 g trans fat, 0 mg cholesterol, 93 mg sodium, 41 g total carbohydrates, 7 g dietary fiber, 17 g sugar, 4 g protein, 257% vitamin A, 187% vitamin C, 15% calcium, 27% iron

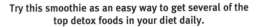

"Think of the top detoxification foods like scrub brushes for your body. They go through your blood, tissues, and organs 'scrubbing out' the harmful stuff, allowing your body to work at peak performance."

Jenna Braddock, Consultant and Sports Dietitian, University of North Florida

See your doctor
Anyone considering going on a fast should consult a physician before embarking on this extreme diet. Prolonged fasting is dangerous and not advised.

Fasting

The oldest and most radical of diets, fasting is the practice of refraining from eating food alongside the sole consumption of water or juice.

The rationale behind a fast is that the total avoidance of food provides a quick weight-loss method. In some cultures, this practice serves as a form of penitence for overindulgence and has religious overtones.

How it works
Without food, blood sugar levels go down as no essential fuel in the form of energy is entering the body. This dip is registered and a neurochemical message is sent to the brain, causing hunger pangs to kick in. During a fast, feelings of hunger come and go as the body is reminding you that you will need to eat at some point. During the first few hours of the fast, the body will obtain energy or glucose either from the glycogen stored in the muscles (only for use by the muscles) or the liver (for use by the rest of the body). This energy reserve lasts for several hours, generally about half a day, or two to three skipped meals. Once used up, and if food does not enter the body, protein from muscle and fat will be broken down and turned to glucose as energy.

Proceed with much caution, if at all
With prolonged fasting, a physical state known as ketosis kicks in. Fasting causes water loss and large amounts of muscle breakdown because it is largely composed of protein. As muscle is broken down, nitrogen is eliminated from the body. Important minerals such as sodium, potassium, and calcium are depleted and this has harmful effects on the body. Low potassium levels, for example, negatively affect the state of the heart and can even be a cause of death during fasting.

The importance of glucose in a healthy functioning body cannot be overstated. The brain consumes the largest amount of glucose, so when blood sugar levels drop, the brain is unable to function properly. As a result, the person may feel confused, dizzy, lightheaded, and have difficulty concentrating. The dieter may feel weak because the muscles are lacking in fuel and the blood is not pumping enough energy to the muscles and the cells. To make up for this decrease in energy, the metabolic rate slows down.

Pros

A quick way of shedding pounds—fat and muscle are used up and water lost.

You don't need to fast for long—it should never exceed a period of two days.

Cons

Once food is re-introduced, the body will gain weight quickly as it replenishes.

Causes some physical discomfort—a complete lack of food will cause you to feel weak and so restrict your activity levels.

Generally not recommended by any dietitians.

After a period of deprivation, the dieter runs the risk of either eating uncontrollably or overeating.

Patients with a heart condition or other illnesses should be very careful or avoid it altogether.

147

Consider a more relaxed approach
In an attempt to moderate the physical consequences resulting from muscle loss, some variations on the fasting method are more of a partial fast and include the consumption of juices. See pages 96–97 for detox diet methods.

Popular diets

Daniel fast
A partial fast that includes fruits, vegetables, and water.

Juice fast diet
Includes raw vegetable and fruit juices and water.

The 5:2 diet
Intermittent fasting diet in which you eat for five days and then eat one quarter of your usual calories for two days.

1 Planning a fast? First check with your physician to make sure you are physically healthy for "no food" for a couple of days. Once given the okay, make sure you fast during days where nothing vigorous, new, or different is scheduled. Try a restful weekend.

2 Do not go on a fast if you have diabetes, heart disease, or any other health condition, or are taking medication. See your physician first for approval, and if obtained, a registered dietitian to help you plan a safe way to fast.

3 Remember: You should never fast for longer than two days.

 sample menu

149 FASTING PLAN
~

You can build up to fasting gradually, over the course of a week. Start by eating a healthy, full three meals a day, then in the final three days:

~

Day 5

BREAKFAST

Cold cereal, milk, banana; wholewheat toast and jam; tea

LUNCH

Vegetable stir-fry with tofu, bok choy, peppers and brown rice; tea

DINNER

Beef barley soup; green salad; fruit salad; tea

~

DAY 6

BREAKFAST

Vanilla yogurt; honeydew melon; tea

LUNCH

Vegetable soup; green salad; tea

DINNER

Miso soup; crackers; green tea

~

DAY 7

Tea and water throughout the day

150 Drink water, and plenty of it

During a fast, the kidneys have to work hard to get rid of the excess waste products with significant water loss. It is vital to drink lots of water during a total fast to avoid toxins accumulating in the blood and promote their elimination through urine. Fasting may give the intestinal tract a rest but the kidneys are overworked and other organs will suffer breakdown for use as energy.

 Do this...

✓ Watch for signs such as thirst, dizziness, shakiness, weakness, chills, lethargy, incoherence, or other physical effects that indicate potential danger.

...Not this

✗ Ignore physical signs of stress and risk a health crisis.

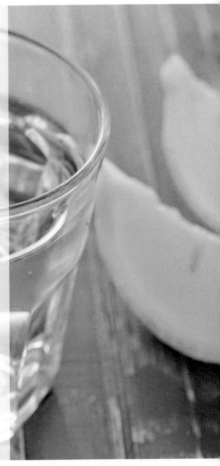

151 Other drinks

Most fasts do not allow consumption of beverages other than water. Try adding a slice of fruit or a berry for flavor—just don't eat it! Some fasts, however, may allow teas, in which case mint and chamomile are sound choices. Coffee, juices, or plant-based smoothies may be permitted in partial fasts.

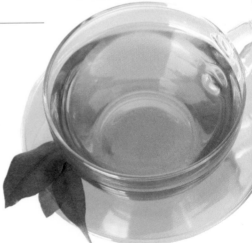

The raw food diet

The raw food diet is a type of diet in which people eat food that is not cooked or processed.

Raw foodists do not eat many, if any, cooked foods because they believe that cooking destroys living plant enzymes that help with digestion and that it reduces vitamins and minerals in food. Common reasons for following this diet include beliefs that it can prevent or cure disease, improve health and energy, and result in weight loss.

What can you eat?

Raw foodists eat at least 70–75% of foods (by weight) raw. Allowed foods include raw fruits, vegetables, nuts, seeds, beans, grains, seaweed, and sprouts. Avoided foods include cooked foods, alcohol, caffeine, and refined sugars. Some people do not eat cereal grains. Many raw foodists are vegetarian or vegan. Some eat unpasteurized dairy foods and raw meats or fish. Strict followers only eat one type of food at a time.

You can heat food to 92–118°F (33–48°C) and the food is still considered raw. Over this temperature, raw foodists believe food changes from living to dead as heat destroys enzymes and vitamins. Instead of cooking, raw foodists use dehydrators, blenders, juicers, soaking, and sprouting to process their foods.

The cooking debate

Our bodies have all the enzymes needed to get nutrition from food. In fact, the plant enzymes in uncooked foods do not even make it through the stomach since they are made up of proteins, which cannot survive stomach acid. Cooking does change the nutrition of some foods and can reduce or improve nutrition. For example, vitamin C can be lost when you cook vegetables in water and B vitamins are lost when manufacturers refine grains. However, your body can more easily absorb lycopene in tomatoes and proteins in eggs when they're cooked. Heat also destroys bacteria and toxins that can cause food-borne illness.

Many testimonials for this diet are from people who previously ate processed "junk" foods. Replacing high-calorie, nutrition-poor processed foods with low-calorie nutrition-rich whole foods could be the reason for the improvements. Testimonials do not provide sufficient valid evidence for the health and safety of a diet.

Pros		Cons	
High in vitamins, minerals, and fiber; low in saturated/trans fats, cholesterol, and added sugars.	Appears to reduce symptoms of rheumatoid arthritis and fibromyalgia.	Not recommended for growing children.	May increase some cardiovascular risk factors, such as lowering HDL (good) cholesterol and increasing homocysteine levels.
May decrease some cardiovascular risk factors, such as reducing blood pressure, cholesterol, and triglyceride levels.	Improved immune system function.	In women, low calories can lead to excessive weight and body-fat loss and result in loss of menstruation.	Increases risk of food-borne illness from bacteria, parasites, toxins, and unpasteurized foods.
Followers have a lower body mass index (BMI) than meat eaters and vegetarians (are less likely to be overweight).	Followers report improved health and better quality of life.	A large amount of misinformation and unproven claims (raw food cures cancer, cooked oils are more fattening than uncooked oils).	
Less time spent in kitchen because of minimal hands-on preparation time.		Followers report being continually hungry.	Lowers bone mass.

1 Interested but don't want to go totally raw? Try eating more salads and fresh, raw fruits and vegetables.

2 Munch on washed crispy snap peas, carrots, celery, asparagus, and mushrooms tossed with chopped herbs and pepper for savory snacks.

3 Mash your favorite berries into a purée and spoon over chopped fruit as a healthy sweetener.

4 To make sure your body gets all the nutrition it needs, take a multivitamin/mineral and work with a registered dietitian.

 153 **RAW FOOD DIET** *sample menu*

~
BREAKFAST

Quinoa soaked overnight in water, topped with bananas, blueberries, cinnamon, and raw honey

Juiced wheatgrass and carrots

~
SNACK

Walnuts, shredded dried coconut, and raisins (or fruit dried in a dehydrator)

~
LUNCH

Sashimi

Seaweed salad

Herbal tea with stevia sweetner

~
SNACK

Homemade salsa (tomatoes, jalapeños, cilantro, onion, lime juice, cayenne)

Raw flax crackers or plantain chips (made with a dehydrator)

~
DINNER

Zucchini "spaghetti" (cut into small strands) topped with tomato sauce (tomatoes, garlic, basil, olive oil, pine nuts, mixed using a blender) and raw-milk cheese

Spinach, strawberry, avocado salad topped with cold-pressed olive oil

~
DESSERT

Chocolate banana "ice cream" (chop frozen bananas and place in food processor with raw cacao powder; blend on high adding water as needed)

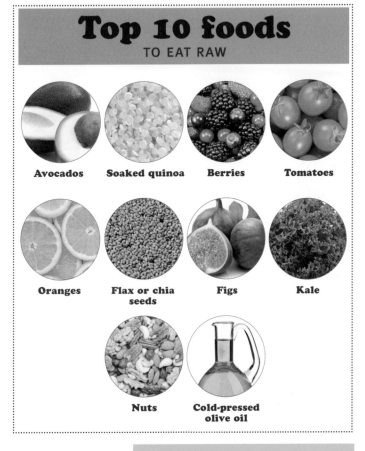
Top 10 foods
TO EAT RAW

Avocados — Soaked quinoa — Berries — Tomatoes — Oranges — Flax or chia seeds — Figs — Kale — Nuts — Cold-pressed olive oil

Popular resources

The RAWvolution Continues: The Living Foods Movement in 150 Natural and Delicious Recipes
By Matt Amsden (Simon & Schuster, Inc./Atria Books, 2013)

www.webmd.com/diet/raw-foods-diet
A useful summary of the diet along with suggestions for further reading.

Living and Raw Foods: www.living-foods.com
The largest community on the Internet dedicated to educating the world about the power of living and raw foods.

"There is not much scientific research on the raw diet, but there are testimonials about improved health and quality of life."

Alexia Lewis, Wellness Dietitian, University of North Florida, and Nutrition Consultant

The vegan diet

When following the vegan diet, people do not eat any foods that come from animal sources.

People may follow a vegan diet for their health, out of a concern for animal welfare or the environment, to reduce the cost of their food, or for religious or cultural reasons.

Vegans do not eat anything that comes from an animal. This includes meat, poultry, and seafood as well as derivative foods such as milk, cheese, butter, yogurt, eggs, mayonnaise, and honey. Strict vegans do not use any products that have come from animals, such as leather, wool, fur, silk, or pearls. There are many animal ingredients in foods that appear to be vegan. To follow a vegan diet, you will have to learn to read food packages to search for ingredients such as lecithin (from eggs), casein (from milk), gelatin (from animals), and lanolin (from sheep).

Not eating any foods that come from animals can sound like a challenge, but with planning, a vegan diet can be nutritionally complete, and for some people, can be a technique for weight loss.

Safety and suitability

A vegan diet is safe and appropriate for any stage of life from infancy through childhood, adulthood, and into the elderly years. In some cases, families may choose to provide children with a lacto-ovo vegetarian (dairy and eggs) diet to facilitate the inclusion of proteins and adequate calories in the diet. It is also safe for pregnant and nursing women. However, not all vegan foods promote health. It depends on the foods that you choose (see opposite).

You can follow a properly planned vegan diet and still have excellent nutrition and health. It is a good idea to talk to your doctor about changing your diet before doing so to determine if there is a need to monitor your levels of iron, vitamin B12, and vitamin D.

Pros		Cons	
Low in saturated fat and cholesterol; high in fiber, folate, vitamins C and E, magnesium, potassium, phytochemicals (plant compounds).	Lower BMI and weight.	Low in vitamins B12 and D, calcium, iron, zinc, omega-3 fatty acids, and possibly low in iodine if not using iodized salt.	Supplementation may be needed for vitamins B12 and D.
Lower total and LDL (bad) cholesterol levels.	Lower blood pressure.	Packaged foods can be high in saturated and trans fats, sodium, and sugar.	Increase in meal-planning time to ensure the diet is providing appropriate nutrition.
Lower risk of cardiovascular disease, hypertension, type 2 diabetes, and certain cancers.	Improved blood sugar control in people with type 2 diabetes.	Must combine foods to get complete proteins (animal products are complete proteins because they contain all essential amino acids; plant foods do not so they must be paired over the course of the day to provide all amino acids).	

1 Use substitutions in cooking and baking, such as ground flaxseed and water instead of eggs.

2 To promote health, eat plenty of plant proteins, grains, fruits, and vegetables.

3 Avoid foods that are fried or high in sugar and sodium, which may be vegan but do not promote health.

4 Eat fortified foods or take a multivitamin/mineral—it takes a lot of planning to get the right mix of nutrition out of your foods.

155   VEGAN PLAN

sample menu

~

BREAKFAST

Toasted oat cereal topped with raisins, sliced almonds, soy milk

Coffee (soy milk and sweetener if desired)

~

SNACK

Roasted chickpeas (see page 35)

~

LUNCH

Hummus wrap (vegan tortilla, hummus, lettuce, tomato, cucumber)

Apple

~

SNACK

Sweet and salty smoothie (chop banana and pineapple, place in food processor with peanut butter and ground flaxseed, blend on high, add water/ice to achieve desired consistency)

~

DINNER

Whole-wheat spaghetti with sauce made from fresh tomatoes, onions, mushrooms, garlic, marinara sauce, silken/soft tofu, basil, oregano, red pepper flakes (blend after cooking if desired)

Garden salad with oil and vinegar

~

DESSERT

Strawberry banana "ice cream" (mash and freeze strawberries and bananas with stevia sweetner)

Popular resources

Becoming Vegan: The Complete Guide to Adopting a Healthy Plant-Based Diet
By Brenda Davis and Vesanto Melina (Book Publishing Company, 2000)

Oldways: http://oldwayspt.org/
Go to: Oldways Resources/Heritage Pyramids/Vegetarian/Vegan Diet and Pyramid

Vegan pyramid

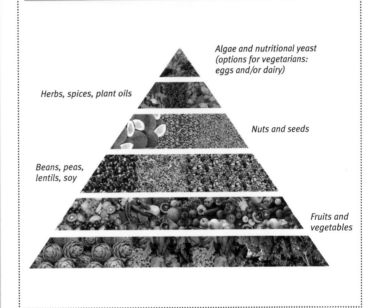

Algae and nutritional yeast (options for vegetarians: eggs and/or dairy)

Herbs, spices, plant oils

Nuts and seeds

Beans, peas, lentils, soy

Fruits and vegetables

156   Quinoa lettuce wraps   serves 12

Ingredients

1½ cups quinoa, rinsed then cooked

1 raw zucchini, diced

1 slice red onion, diced

2 carrots, diced

1 large stalk celery, diced

Handful of chopped walnuts

Handful of raisins

Red wine vinegar, to taste

Black pepper, to taste

Romaine lettuce leaves, rinsed

Directions

1. Mix all ingredients except the last three together.
2. Add red wine vinegar and black pepper in small increments until the dish has a flavor you enjoy.
3. Serve a spoonful of the quinoa mixture onto the raw romaine lettuce leaves and wrap up.

Nutrition per serving (1 wrap): 66 calories, 2 g fat, 18 mg sodium, 10 g carbohydrate, 2 g fiber, 3 g sugar, 2 g protein

The DASH diet

Dietary Approaches to Stop Hypertension (DASH) can help prevent or manage high blood pressure, and provide a balanced diet appropriate for anyone.

The DASH diet increases servings of foods with nutrients that lower blood pressure. Specifically, the diet provides you with less sodium (salt), saturated fat, and cholesterol, and more potassium, calcium, magnesium, and fiber. The DASH diet provides specific numbers of servings from food groups (see below). It encourages you to eat 27% of your calories from fats with 6% being saturated fats, 18% of your calories from protein, and 55% from carbohydrate.

You have flexibility to choose your foods, as long as you stay within the guidelines—the diet gives you a number of servings from different food groups to eat every day.

Scientific research
Researchers used the DASH diet, previously called the combination diet,

to investigate the effect of different diets on blood pressure. The initial study in 1997 recruited 412 American adults with high blood pressure. It compared the typical Western diet to the DASH diet and different levels of sodium. The researchers found the DASH diet—especially when combined with lower sodium—reduced blood pressure. Since that time, many researchers have studied the diet. They have found that is it effective in lowering blood pressure; lowering total cholesterol, LDL cholesterol, and triglycerides; and increasing HDL cholesterol. It also reduces risk for cardiovascular disease and may be helpful in managing type 2 diabetes.

In addition, The National Heart, Lung, and Blood Institute of the U.S. National Institutes of Health studied diets to see if they had an effect on hypertension and found that DASH did lower blood pressure.

The DASH diet promotes good health and healthy attitudes towards food and eating. It is a great way to decrease your calorie intake. If you are concerned about your heart health and blood pressure and you are looking for a non-restrictive well-balanced diet, the DASH diet is right for you.

If you eat 2,000 calories a day, then you should eat:

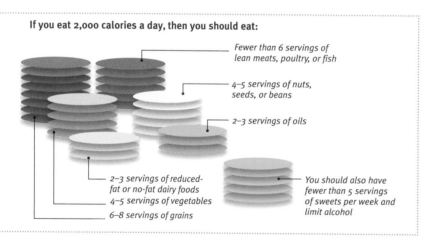

- Fewer than 6 servings of lean meats, poultry, or fish
- 4–5 servings of nuts, seeds, or beans
- 2–3 servings of oils
- 2–3 servings of reduced-fat or no-fat dairy foods
- 4–5 servings of vegetables
- 6–8 servings of grains
- You should also have fewer than 5 servings of sweets per week and limit alcohol

Pros		Cons	
High in fruits, vegetables, fiber; low in saturated and trans fats, sodium, added sugars.	High in potassium, calcium, and vitamins D and B12.	Increase in food preparation time (not relying on packaged or convenience products).	Increase in cost (purchasing fresh fruits and vegetables).
Does not restrict or avoid any food groups.	You can modify it for special needs such as vegetarian/vegan, gluten-free, etc.	Eating in some restaurants may be difficult (typically high in sodium and fat).	Flavor may be lacking at first due to using less salt, but taste buds will adjust.
Promotes a lifestyle approach instead of a dieting approach.			

1 It is recommended to do 30 minutes per day of moderate exercise, alongside the diet plan.

2 Does 8–10 servings of fruits and vegetables a day seem like too much? Start slowly. Identify a meal or snack that typically does not include a fruit or vegetable and find a way to include it. Continue adding to meals and snacks over several weeks.

3 All the foods are readily available from a supermarket and/or grocery store, so shop easily but wisely—see Shopping for vegetables and Shopping for fruit on pages 48–51.

4 To avoid becoming bored with your diet, pick up a fruit or vegetable that you have never tried before.

Popular resources

The DASH Diet Eating Plan: dashdiet.org
The ultimate resource, including related articles, book lists, recipes, and FAQs.

· **The DASH Diet Weight Loss Plan**
By Marla Heller (Grand Central Life & Style, 2012)

Top 5 foods
FOR THE DASH DIET

| Low-fat yogurt | Apricots | Beans | Kale | Popcorn |

---

 158 CHICKEN RATATOUILLE — serves **4**

Ingredients

1 tbsp vegetable oil

4 chicken breast halves, skinned, boned, fat removed, and cubed

2 zucchini, thinly sliced

1 small eggplant, cubed

1 onion, thinly sliced

1 green pepper, chopped

½ lb (230 g) fresh mushrooms, sliced

1 can whole tomatoes, cut up

clove garlic, minced

1½ tsp dried basil

1 tbsp fresh parsley

black pepper

Directions

1. Heat the oil in a skillet. Add the chicken and sauté for 3 minutes, or until lightly browned.

2. Add zucchini, eggplant, onion, green pepper, and mushrooms. Cook for 15 minutes, stirring occasionally.

3. Add tomatoes, garlic, basil, parsley, and pepper; stir and continue cooking for 5 minutes, or until the chicken is tender.

Serving size: 1½ cups
266 calories per serving

---

 159 DASH PLAN — sample menu

~
BREAKFAST
Egg-white omelet cooked in trans-fat-free margarine with tomatoes, broccoli, and bell peppers

Whole-wheat toast topped with mashed strawberries

Coffee or tea with skim milk
~
SNACK
Apple with peanut butter
~
LUNCH
Cottage cheese with walnuts, peaches, and pineapple on whole-wheat crackers
~
DINNER
Chicken stir-fry (zucchini, peppers, onion, etc.) cooked with canola oil, served over brown rice

Edamame and corn salad
~
DESSERT
Yogurt parfait with strawberries and sliced almonds, sprinkled with cocoa powder and cinnamon

The Paleo diet

The Paleo diet is based on the idea that we should eat like our paleolithic ancestors to prevent the onset of today's chronic diseases.

Never go foraging for wild foods without adequate knowledge, skill, and permission!

Eat like the cavemen ate with plenty of meat, poultry, eggs, seafood, vegetables, fruit, honey, and nuts, but no grains (bread, cereal, rice, pasta, oatmeal, cookies, cakes, pies, pastries, muffins, etc.), beans, dairy foods, refined sugars, caffeine, or alcohol. There are several proclaimed health benefits to this diet, and proponents of the diet argue that our ancient ancestors were largely unaffected by "diseases of affluence" such as heart diseases, type 2 diabetes, and obesity. However, the common lifespan during that time was about 35 to 40 years, so others argue that people didn't live long enough to get these "modern-era" chronic diseases. Also, in reality there was no one Paleo diet, because people lived in many different regions throughout the world and were limited to choices available in their environment.

The science behind the diet

The diet fits best into the category of low-carbohydrate high-protein diets. The omission of dairy products and grains may be its most controversial feature. While the diet also promotes whole foods versus processed foods, nutrients that may be limited by dairy and grain restrictions include calories, calcium, vitamin D, B vitamins, fiber, iron, magnesium, and selenium. To date, there is limited to fair evidence that this diet is effective. The diet may also be associated with increased food expense, especially for those buying only grass-fed meats and organic fruits and vegetables.

Beneficial aspects of the diet when compared to current nutritional issues such as obesity and related chronic diseases include potential restriction of calories, carbohydrate, sugar, and salt, and increased consumption of fruits and vegetables, seafood, and nuts.

As you can see, this diet requires major changes for most people and the increased cost may be a deterrent. However, those who adopt this diet tend to be very positive about how they feel and the potential for weight control they experience. So, eating like our cave ancestors did is difficult, requires determination, and may not actually be feasible for you, but many seem to find adopting the hunter-gatherer mentality associated with the Paleo diet is certainly a conversation starter!

> "The Paleo diet may be tough at first for those who have trouble controlling carbohydrate intake from grains and sweets. But, after a period of adjustment, the diet may be healthier and more helpful in weight control due to the elimination of those food categories.

Catherine Christie, Associate Dean and Professor, University of North Florida

Pros		Cons	
Proclaimed benefits include weight loss; reduction in body fat; improved muscle growth, glucose control, and insulin sensitivity; and lowered risk of heart disease.	Fewer calories and carbohydrates; less sugar and salt; more fruits, vegetables, seafood, nuts.	Limited evidence that this diet is effective for weight loss and prevention of diseases of affluence.	Grocery costs and time spent shopping are likely to increase when sourcing specialist foods.
Promotes whole foods over processed foods.	Can be an interesting lifestyle choice, enabling you to learn about the diet of your ancestors.	Restriction of dairy produce can lead to deficiencies.	Requires extensive lifestyle changes and plenty of determination.

1 Try the diet for a short time, if it helps you kick-start your weight loss.

2 Focus on large quantities of fresh fruits and vegetables to provide fiber, which is missing due to the limitation of grains.

3 As a rule of thumb: if you can't hunt or pick it, don't eat it!

4 While following the plan, it is advisable to increase physical activity and drink lots of fresh water.

---

161 **PALEO PLAN**
~
sample menu

BREAKFAST
Broiled cod with sliced tomato
Melon cubes
~
LUNCH
8 oz (200g) baked free-range chicken
Salad with lettuce, carrots, cucumbers, tomatoes, walnuts, and lemon juice
~
DINNER
8 oz (200 g) sirloin roast
Steamed cauliflower and broccoli
Salad with mixed greens, cabbage, tomatoes, avocado, almonds, onions, and lemon juice
Mixed berries
~
SNACKS
Fresh fruit or vegetables

Top 10 foods
TO EAT RAW

Avocado

Free-range poultry

Fruit

Grass-fed lean beef

Grass-fed lean lamb

Non-starchy vegetables

Omega-3-rich eggs

Tea

Unsalted nuts

Wild fish and shellfish

 162

Questions to ask yourself when considering the Paleo diet:
• Do you enjoy grains? Do you like dairy products? Are you willing to give them up permanently?
• Can you think of other options, such as moderating the amounts of these foods?
• Are you at potential risk for some health conditions, and how might such a plan impact you? Do you have a family history of osteoporosis? Are you prone to anemia or planning on getting pregnant, when iron intake is very important?
• Is it difficult for you to get some of the foods required on the Paleo plan either geographically or financially?
• Do you live alone? How might following the diet impact others?
• How easily will it fit your lifestyle, such as eating at work or eating out?

Popular resources

The Paleo Diet Revised
By Loren Cordain (Houghton Mifflin Harcourt, 2010)

Living Paleo for Dummies
By Melissa Joulwan and Kellyann Petrucci (For Dummies, 2012)

See your doctor
If you are thinking about trying a Paleo plan, see your doctor to be sure your health conditions will not be aggravated by eliminating some important food groups from your diet.

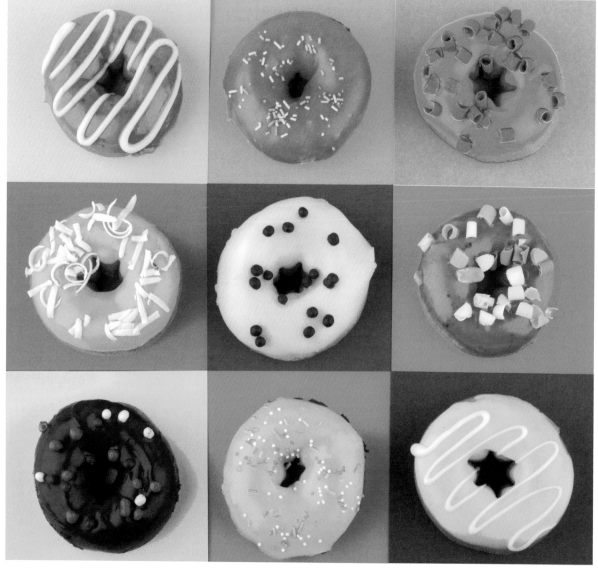

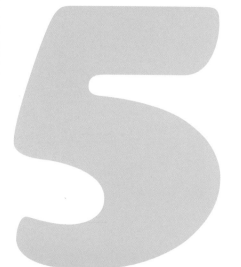

Where there's a high amount of sugar, there's usually a high amount of fats—especially saturated fats—lurking within as well. So that's two good reasons to steer clear!

Ways to overcome sugar cravings

When it comes to food-related cravings, the dreaded sugar craving is at the top of the list for most people. Fortunately, there are ways to overcome the urge to splurge.

Empty calories

First of all, let's look at how pointless eating added sugar really is. Refined white sugar (the sort used in manufactured foods) is a carbohydrate that provides energy but none of the desirable extra nutrition supplied by other carbohydrates, such as whole grains. So while sugar might not actually be "bad" for you, it's not good for you either, and eating too much of it certainly isn't. Studies are currently being carried out to establish whether it is addictive.

Break the habit

Hard though it is to imagine as you reach for yet another cookie, it only takes 21 days to break a habit. Easy as that? Almost! If you can discipline yourself to follow a holistic plan that includes eating plant-based foods at regular intervals, washed down with plenty of water, as well as engaging in meditation, deep breathing, and gentle exercise every day, with a good night's sleep to round it all off, you'll find that your sugar cravings will be diminished considerably. Even those infamous premenstrual give-me-chocolate-or-I'll-scream cravings, endured both by women and their long-suffering nearest and dearest, simply vanish!

Try baking at home with alternative healthy ingredients. Experimenting with color can further entice your appetite for health.

Manage your sugar consumption

Once you've broken the habit, you'll still need to keep your sugar intake under control:

Never shop when you're hungry. When your blood sugar is low, your instinct is to reach for generous quantities of anything sweet.

Include plenty of healthy fats in your diet. Illogical though it might seem to include "plenty" and "fat" in the same sentence, fats actually inform your brain when you're full—unlike sugar, which simply encourages you to keep eating even to the point of feeling nauseous.

Learn a few savvy tricks for including things in your diet that have a sweet taste to satisfy your taste buds.
For example:
• Snack on a few almonds, which are naturally sweet, filling, and full of nutrients.
• Add a pinch of Ceylon cinnamon to oatmeal instead of sugar—not only is it a warm, sweet spice but it also contains traces of coumarin, a compound that stabilizes blood sugar levels.
• Learn a new way of baking, using ingredients such as sweet potatoes, beets, and ground almonds to provide sweetness. You'll soon find that manufactured or even home-baked sugar-laden products taste far too sweet.
• Nominate one day a week as your ritual "cheat" day (if cheating appeals to your psychology) or a "treat" day (if treating feels better than cheating). Find a special location in which to cheat/treat—a lovely café that serves home-baked goodies in an environment that appeals to you. Perhaps take a half-hour walk first, just enough to release endorphins but not so energetic as to make you ravenous, then go and enjoy ONE special sugary treat. Afterward, walk away and look forward to next week!

Graze your way through the day

Forget about "trying not to eat between meals." Sensible snacking will keep your blood sugar levels stable and you will be far less likely to binge on something sweet if you eat breakfast, a mid-morning snack, lunch, a mid-afternoon snack, and dinner. To maintain a stable weight, allow 500 calories for the main meals and 250 calories for each of the snacks (or increase or decrease the amount, depending on your daily calorie requirement for your gender/age/weight/activity level). Choose your snacks wisely: this is not a legitimate opportunity to eat a pastry in the morning and a chocolate bar in the afternoon! See pages 34–35 for healthy snack ideas.

Eat mindfully

This is perhaps one of the most important things you can do for your health, and certainly in terms of overcoming sugar cravings. Mindfulness is an ancient Buddhist practice that is now being applied to many aspects of life, and it is exactly what it suggests: keeping your awareness in the "here and now" so that you are mindful of everything you do. If you usually eat on autopilot, unconscious of what's going into your mouth as you catch up on reading emails at your desk or flop in front of the TV, try instead to focus completely on what you're eating. Be mindful of every bite, and your brain will register satisfaction.

Head off stress

Sugar cravings are often triggered by stress, which causes physiological changes in the body that are exacerbated by sugar, rather than relieved by it. Arm yourself against stress by eating a diet rich in stress-busting foods, such as broccoli, fish, almonds, bananas—and chocolate. Not the cheap, mass-produced type, but a good-quality very dark chocolate rich in polyphenols, which repair damage caused by stress hormones.

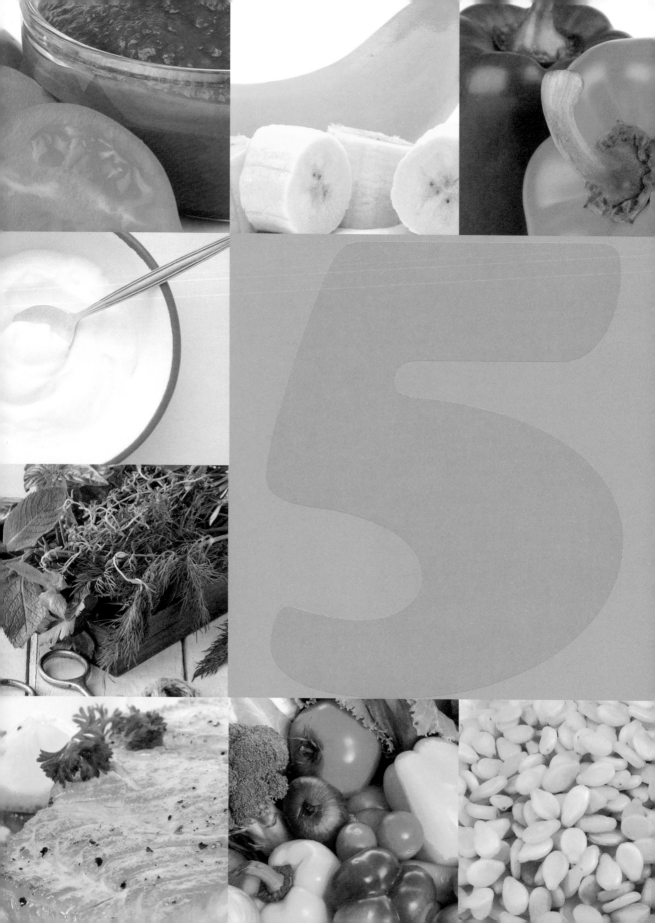

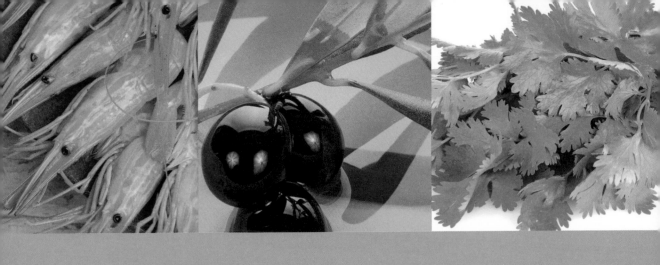

Special
health
concerns

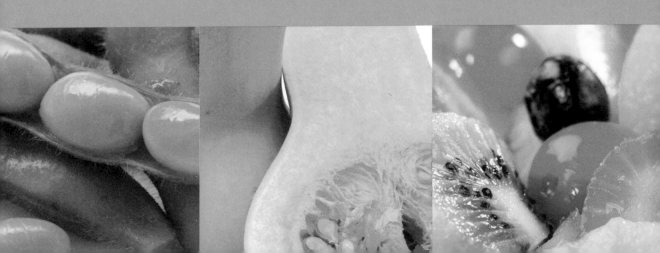

Specific dietary requirements

You can eat healthy, delicious foods even when you have special health needs. With the right knowledge, you can easily navigate your daily eating with success.

A person's diet is determined by many factors. Age, gender, health concerns, and lifestyle all play a role in why you should eat a certain way. If you need a special eating plan for any reason, embrace it and know that you can enjoy a healthy and delicious diet with practice and time.

The most common reasons people need a specialized diet are:
• When the body has higher-than-usual nutrient demands, such as times of accelerated growth or related needs, as in the first year of life, during pre-teen and teen years, in pregnancy, or during sport training.
• When trying to avoid or treat a specific health condition, such as an allergy or heart disease.
• When lifestyle changes mean you require less energy, such as when you age.

Reactions to food

Food sensitivity or intolerance is another area where specialized diets are needed. Food intolerance is different from an allergy. An allergy is the result of the body's immune system reacting to a food—even a small amount has the potential to be fatal. But a food intolerance or sensitivity is usually a gastrointestinal response to a food. With a food intolerance or sensitivity, you may not require total elimination of foods that you struggle with and may be able to eat and enjoy a small amount of the food. Knowing exactly what is going on with your body will help you make the best diet decisions.

Many of today's major causes of death are lifestyle related. If you have a risk of heart disease, diabetes, high blood pressure, or kidney disease in your family history, eating in a certain way can help to significantly reduce that risk. In fact, a healthy diet has been shown to help reverse certain diseases or, even better, prevent them altogether. Even though it is difficult to make some changes, you can be certain that they will make a big difference to your long-term health.

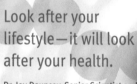

Look after your lifestyle—it will look after your health.

Dr. Joy Dauncey, Senior Scientist and Adviser in Nutritional and Biomedical Sciences, University of Cambridge, U.K.

 Do this...

✓ Get antioxidants from foods, such as resveratrol (which may lower risk of heart disease) from red and purple foods such as grapes or pomegranates. That way you will get many other antioxidants at the same time.

 ...Not this

✗ Get the same antioxidant from a pill or think that you can only get it from red wine.

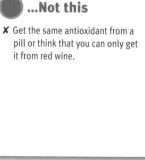

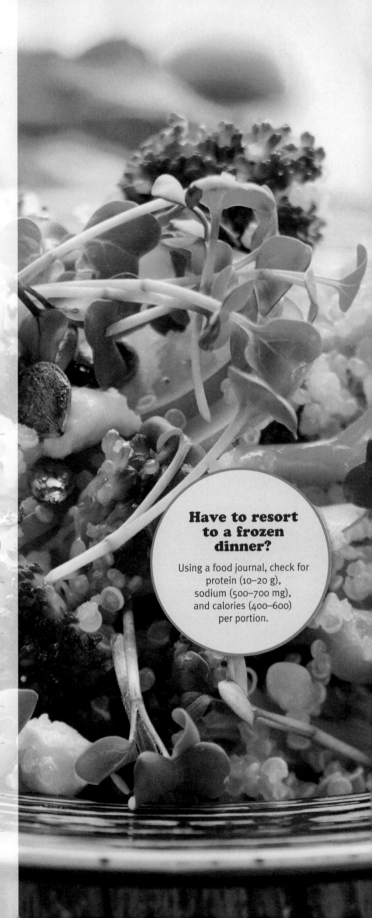

Easy preventive measures

Evaluate why and if you really need a special diet. Often people are mostly influenced by dieting trends instead of considering what will truly benefit their health.

Add flavor to your meat, fish, or poultry without calories or salt by "reducing" flavored vinegar and using that instead of gravy or sauce (for example, heat balsamic vinegar in a pan until some water evaporates, or produces a "reduction").

Increase your folic acid intake by making your smoothies with orange juice instead of water.

Increase your iron intake by cooking in cast-iron pans.

Eat to prevent cancer by emphasizing cruciferous vegetables. Want an easy way to find them? Look for veggies that have leaves that "cross or overlap" each other (members of the cabbage family, such as cabbage, cauliflower, broccoli, Brussels sprouts, bok choy, etc.).

Your place in the life cycle

Understanding where you or your loved ones are in your life cycle and health needs will enable you to make the best diet choices for long-term health and vitality. You should always take into account your personal needs and concerns before deciding to jump on the latest eating trend. A simple awareness of growth patterns and physiology can help you make the best choices for your optimal health. For example:

• Babies approximately triple in weight and double in height in the first year of life, and this is why they need to be fed so often during the day.

• Girls need to increase their iron intake when they begin menstruation.

• Pregnant women ideally need to consume adequate amounts of folic acid before they get pregnant.

• Men need lycopene, which is found in tomato and tomato products and may help prevent prostate cancer.

• As you age you need fewer calories but the same amount, or more, of some nutrients, which means your diet has to be more "nutrient dense."

• Some athletes think they need a lot more protein and fewer carbohydrates than they actually do.

Have to resort to a frozen dinner?

Using a food journal, check for protein (10–20 g), sodium (500–700 mg), and calories (400–600) per portion.

Diabetes

Living with diabetes can be a challenge—you have to learn to balance your meals and make the healthiest food choices possible.

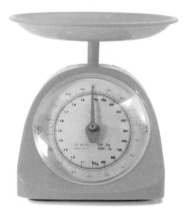

Living with diabetes may leave you constantly asking yourself, "What *can* I eat?" There is not a universal nutrition approach for people with diabetes; however, it is possible to give a few basic tips to help you make positive choices.

When you find out you have diabetes, you may feel that knowing what to eat is confusing. Once you become comfortable with making appropriate choices throughout the day, you will realize that you can incorporate a variety of foods into your meal plan, manage your blood sugar, and enjoy a healthy life.

> A steady and correct amount of healthy carbohydrates throughout the day will help stabilize blood sugar levels.

What can you drink?

Don't forget that the calorie-containing beverages you drink also raise your blood glucose levels and may cause weight gain if they contribute to excess calories. Drink zero-calorie or very low calorie drinks such as:
• Water
• Unsweetened teas and coffee
• Diet soda
• No-calorie drink mixes

Avoid sugary drinks that raise blood glucose levels and can provide hundreds of calories in just one serving. For example:
• One 12 fl oz (350 ml) can of regular soda: about 150 calories and 40 g of carbohydrate (or 10 teaspoons of sugar)
• One 8 fl oz (240 ml) glass of fruit punch or other sugary fruit drinks: about 100 calories (or more) and 30 g of carbohydrate (or 7–8 teaspoons of sugar). Alcoholic beverages are generally not recommended if you have diabetes, unless approved by your physician.

Quick guide to carbs

One serving of carbohydrate equals 15 g. Examples include:
• 1 slice white or whole-wheat bread
• ¾ cup unsweetened dry cereal
• ½ cup cooked beans or corn
• ⅓ cup cooked pasta or rice
• ⅛ of 12 inch (30 cm) thin pizza (crust)

Remember that 15 g is one carbohydrate serving and about 4–5 g of sugar are one teaspoon of sugar. If the label says 15 g of carbohydrate and 10 g of sugar, two thirds of those carbohydrates per serving are sugar!

Check this out

American Diabetes Association:
www.diabetes.org
Information on food and fitness for diabetics.

Eating for diabetes

1 Emphasize whole grains and avoid the processed white flour-based products, especially the ones with added sugars. Look at the Nutrition Facts label and try to select cereals and grains with at least 3 g of fiber per serving—not all whole-grain items are high in fiber.

2 It is important to choose grains that are rich in vitamins—especially B vitamins—and contain minerals, fiber, and phytochemicals. Look for quantities on the Nutrition Facts label.

3 Protein foods are an important part of a balanced diabetes meal plan. Plan a meal with balance and moderation, which means about 2–5 oz (55–140 g) of meat, poultry, or fish.

4 Avoid sugary drinks, saturated fats, and trans fats. Steer clear of processed snack foods.

Top 5 foods in main groups

 169

Fats and carbs in protein

Meat, poultry, and fish do not contain carbohydrates but do contain protein and fat, which can help with satiety (the feeling of fullness) and do not raise blood glucose levels. But, one area to watch for in meat and poultry is the amount of saturated and total fats. For meat substitutes, check whether the product contains carbohydrates. This will be important for you to know so you can include that amount into your carbohydrate meal plan and your total intake. This is important for managing your blood sugar levels.

170

Plating up the protein

Make one quarter of your plate high-protein foods, such as a small chicken breast or 3–4 oz (85–110 g) of lean beef or pork loin, one quarter from whole grains, and the other half from vegetables and fruits. When you have a mixed dish or casserole that includes a starch and meat (such as lasagna or a shepherd's pie), that equates to about half the plate. The other half of your plate should be made up of non-starchy vegetables.

 171

Remember dairy

Dairy products provide you with good-quality protein and are also an easy way to get calcium in your diet. Among the better choices in dairy products are:
• Fat-free or low-fat milk (1%)
• Plain non-fat regular/light or Greek yogurt
• Low or non-fat cheeses

Low-fat Greek yogurt

Whole grains (rich in vitamins, minerals, fiber, and phytochemicals)

Brown rice | Whole oats/oatmeal | Buckwheat | Millet | Quinoa

Starchy vegetables (great sources of vitamins, minerals, and fiber)

Butternut squash | Corn | Green peas | Parsnips | Plantain

Protein foods (lowest in saturated fats)

White fish | Skinless chicken or turkey breast | Pork loin | Egg whites | Dried beans, lentils, peas, legumes

Fish (high in omega-3)

Tuna | Salmon | Herring | Mackerel | Rainbow trout

Shellfish (high in omega-3)

Clams | Crab | Lobster | Scallops | Shrimp

Monounsaturated fats (can help lower cholesterol)

   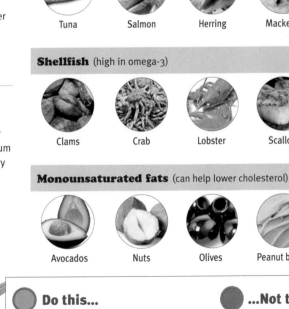

Avocados | Nuts | Olives | Peanut butter | Sesame seeds

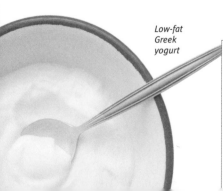

Do this...
✓ Estimate how much of the carbohydrates in each meal are appropriate for you.
✓ Get plenty of fiber from beans, fruits, vegetables, nuts, seeds, and grains, such as brown rice or whole-wheat breads.

...Not this
✗ Get most of the carbohydrates in your meal from breads, crackers, or pasta made from refined white flour.
✗ Have a diet that is primarily refined carbohydrates or concentrated sweets, such as white bread or cakes.

High blood pressure

You can still eat delicious foods when you have high blood pressure—low in salt does not mean low in flavor.

Blood pressure is the force or pressure of blood against artery walls and is recorded as two numbers. The systolic pressure number is the pressure when the heart beats and the diastolic pressure is when the heart relaxes between beats. Did you automatically assume that a diagnosis of high blood pressure meant a life of bland, boring food? Well, the good news is that when you cut back on sodium or salt, you actually learn to enjoy the wide range of flavors of foods, instead of adding flavor with salt.

A low-salt diet means limiting the amount of table salt (sodium chloride) added to your food, whereas a low-sodium diet means limiting table salt and the sodium found in other forms (for example, monosodium glutamate). Remember that fresh foods will offer the least amount of salt compared to the same foods that are canned and processed, such as high-salt canned vegetables. Look to buy fresh produce and frozen alternatives.

Store-bought, restaurant-cooked, homemade
Food labels list foods as low-, lower-, reduced-, or no-salt-added versions. At home, you have more control over the amount of salt you add to food, so salt can be reduced or not included at all in homemade dishes. Also, when eating out, ask how the meals are prepared. For example, a potato could be rolled in salt before it is cooked, so ask questions about how items are prepared and cooked, and ask for a salt-free version of your dish if necessary.

Lifestyle changes
Not only is watching your salt and sodium intake important, but there are other ways you can manage high blood pressure like losing weight, adopting the Dietary Approaches to Stop Hypertension (DASH) eating plan (see pages 104–105), regular aerobic exercise (see pages 36–41), and moderating alcohol consumption (see pages 86–87).

> It is important to learn to read labels, taking special care to look for and read sodium levels.

Corinne Labyak, Assistant Professor, University of North Florida

You can still enjoy your favorite foods with just a few slight twists. Put down the salt shaker and read the labels for sodium content. You will find your taste buds might take a few weeks to adjust but it's worth it in the end.

172

Effects of alcohol
Although a small amount of alcohol such as wine may help lower blood pressure, if you don't drink, don't start just for the intent of lowering blood pressure (losing weight or lowering sodium intake are better ways to do this). Alcoholic beverages in large amounts may worsen (increase) your blood pressure. This may occur with two, three, or more drinks consumed at one event. Alcoholic beverages also contain calories, which may contribute to weight gain. If you are taking medications for high blood pressure, it is important to ask your doctor if alcohol interferes with your medicine's effectiveness or increases its side-effects.

Food ingredient label red flags:
salt, sodium chloride, sodium, monosodium glutamate (MSG), sodium nitrate, sodium alginate, and sodium bicarbonate

Better to make it fresh!

173 Five ways to reduce your salt intake and lower your blood pressure

1 Avoid foods that are listed as pickled, cured, smoked, or broth.

2 Check the label and select the low-, reduced-sodium, or no-salt-added versions of foods.

3 Choose fresh or frozen fruits and vegetables.

4 Identify high-sodium foods within your diet and read labels to find lower-sodium replacements.

5 Have unsalted versions of your favorite nuts as a snack.

Tempt the taste buds	
Like savory? Instead of salt:	**Like spicy or hot? Instead of salt:**
Add cilantro with tomatoes	Add cayenne pepper to popcorn
Add balsamic vinegar to grilled vegetables	Add jalapeños on top of a baked potato or to your homemade chili
Add dill weed or rosemary to rice	Add a dash of Tabasco (pepper) sauce to your soups or stews

Four ways to manage stress

Whether stress causes long-term high blood pressure is uncertain, but there is no doubt that behaviors linked to stress (overeating, smoking, drinking, insomnia) contribute to the condition; in the short-term, stress causes your blood pressure to peak, which over time can culminate in a high blood pressure condition. Try these ways for combatting the stress in your life.

1 Avoid situations, people, topics, or things that upset you. Walk away from the stressful situation.

2 Alter the way you respond. Instead of yelling, try a 10-minute "cooling off" period before explaining what upset you.

3 Adapt to situations you cannot control. Determine how you can manage the issue and find a positive aspect to the situation.

4 Accept things that cannot be controlled or changed, forgive, and let go of grudges, old anger, disappointment, or hostility.

Easy meal

Marinate chicken in lemon juice and dried parsley that contains no sodium. Grill it for 6–8 minutes on each side and serve with a baked potato with 1 tablespoon of unsalted butter and a side salad with your favorite oil and vinegar.

Cooking with a grill or ridged griddle pan not only creates attractive, tasty lines on meat—it also prevents the meat from sitting in grease while it cooks.

Do this...

✓ Make your own soups to keep sodium content to a minimum.

✓ Add fresh seasonings to your meals. Consider growing your own in window boxes or in your garden.

✓ Keep stress at bay with a soothing herbal tea such as chamomile.

...Not this

✗ Buy commercial soups. Read the label—most are high in salt or sodium.

✗ Add salt substitutes or commercial seasonings. Some contain potassium chloride and need to be avoided by people with kidney disease or certain medications for your kidneys, heart, or liver.

✗ Reach for caffeine-fueled tea or coffee when you are feeling under pressure.

Top salt-busters

Fresh herbs

Vinegars

Lemon

Spices

Heart disease

Eating certain foods can reduce your risk of coronary heart disease or help you manage existing heart disease.

Heart disease is a health concern worldwide. According to the American Heart Association and the European Heart Network, the number of people dying from heart disease is decreasing, but it is still the leading cause of death. Heart disease may be a result of damage to blood vessels from a build-up of plaque (coronary heart disease), from bacteria (rheumatic heart disease), or from being born with congenital heart disease.

The good news is that you can eat in a way that keeps your heart more healthy. Nutrition also affects conditions that increase risk of heart disease (high blood pressure, high cholesterol, diabetes, and overweight/obesity). Manage your total caloric intake to avoid the excessive calories that lead to overweight/obesity. Limit your intake of saturated fats which are found in meats, coconut, whole-fat milk or cheese, and cholesterol, which is found in animal sources such as meat or egg yolks.

Recovering from surgery

If you have had heart bypass surgery manage your recovery to help decrease the possibilities of complications. Make sure you take the prescribed medications, monitor symptoms, and eat a heart-smart diet. This includes at least five servings of fresh fruits and vegetables, and low-salt, low-saturated-fat, and low-cholesterol foods.

People recover in different ways from heart bypass surgery so don't compare your recovery to anyone else's recovery in terms of length of time or abilities.

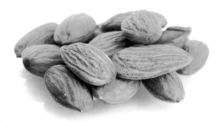

Get jumping to get that heart pumping. Don't forget to exercise today.

176

Eat the right fats

Trans fats are in packaged foods and bakery items, and can appear in foods as "partially hydrogenated" oils. To replace saturated fats with unsaturated fats, choose liquid over solid oils. Add foods like avocado, almonds, and canola oil, which are high in unsaturated fats. Include more meatless meals; many meats are high in saturated fat and cholesterol.

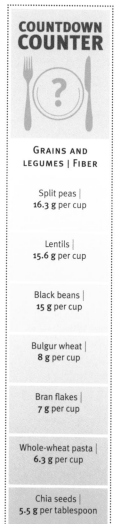

COUNTDOWN COUNTER

?

GRAINS AND LEGUMES | FIBER

Split peas |
16.3 g per cup

Lentils |
15.6 g per cup

Black beans |
15 g per cup

Bulgur wheat |
8 g per cup

Bran flakes |
7 g per cup

Whole-wheat pasta |
6.3 g per cup

Chia seeds |
5.5 g per tablespoon

Almonds |
4 g per ½ cup

Flaxseed meal |
3.8 g per
2 tablespoons

Brown rice |
3.5 g per cup

177 **Follow these guidelines for a heart-healthy diet**

1 Enjoy at least 4–5 cups of whole fruits and vegetables a day. These are full of fiber and heart-healthy vitamins and minerals such as potassium and magnesium. They are low in calories, which means they fill you up without increasing your weight.

2 Eat at least two servings of fish (3–4 ounces/85–110 g) a week. Fish is heart-healthy because it includes omega-3 unsaturated fat. Choose fatty fish like salmon, mackerel, or herring. If you don't eat fish, eat other sources of omega-3 fats such as walnuts, canola oil, or ground flaxseed. Fish is also a lower-calorie, lower-fat protein than meat.

3 Focus on fiber-rich foods. Women should eat 21–25 g and men 30–38 g of fiber a day. Choose foods that have at least 3 g (ideally over 5 g) of fiber per serving. Eat plenty of whole-grain foods and don't just limit yourself to whole-wheat bread and pasta—try brown rice, popcorn, quinoa, and millet.

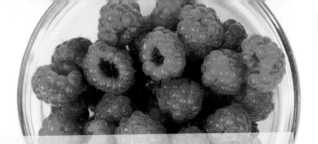

Raspberries are low in fat and have high levels of polyphenols, which help reduce heart disease risk.

Cholesterol watch

A fatty substance produced naturally by the liver, cholesterol only becomes a problem for the body when the levels are too high. Eating the wrong types of foods can cause levels to reach potentially harmful levels, clogging arteries and putting you at risk of major heart disease. Try to minimize foods that are high in saturated fat, such as eggs, meats, and dairy products with fat, butter, or lard.

Food	Cholesterol
1 egg	185 mg
3 oz (85 g) ground beef, 80% lean	77 mg
1 glass regular milk	24 mg
1 tsp butter	10 mg
1 glass skim milk	5 mg
1 oz (30 g) shredded coconut	0 mg

COUNTDOWN COUNTER

FRUIT AND VEGETABLES | FIBER

Artichoke, cooked | 10.3 g

Green peas, cooked | 8.8 g per cup

Raspberries | 8 g per cup

Avocado, half | 6.7 g

Pear | 5.5 g

Broccoli | 5.1 g per cup

Turnip greens | 5 g per cup

Sweet potato | 4.8 g

Apple | 4 g

Corn, cooked | 4 g per cup

Raisins | 3 g per ½ cup

Top 10 foods
FOR HEART HEALTH

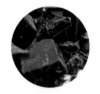
Dark chocolate

Ground flaxseed

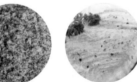
Salmon and other fatty fish

Olive and canola oil

Nuts

Avocado

Red grapes

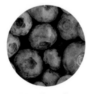
Blueberries

Green tea

Beans

4 To reduce blood pressure, choose **fresh foods** instead of packaged or canned foods. If you use canned foods, rinse to reduce sodium. Season your dishes with spices, herbs, or lemon juice.

5 Limit sugar-sweetened drinks to less than 500 calories a week. Added sugars are associated with increased heart disease risk, possibly because they increase weight and triglycerides. Make soda, candy, desserts, and sugar-sweetened foods a treat instead of a daily part of your diet.

6 Avoid trans fats, replace saturated fats with unsaturated fats, and limit dietary cholesterol to 300 mg a day.

Potato chips and the alternatives

Potato chips tantalize your taste buds and test your willpower. The combination of carbs, fat, and salt is irresistible—let's face it, once you've started, it's virtually impossible to stop.

The percentages of the recommended daily value shown below are typical for a 1-oz (30-g)—tiny!—serving of sea-salt flavor natural potato chips, the least processed type of chip. Frightening, isn't it?

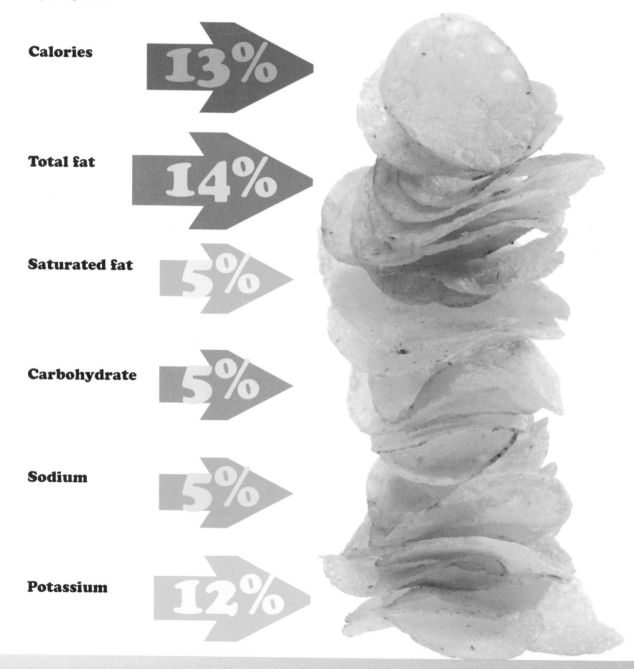

Calories 13%

Total fat 14%

Saturated fat 5%

Carbohydrate 5%

Sodium 5%

Potassium 12%

Chip cravings tend to fall into two categories: a little something to nibble on while you relax with a glass of wine or lager, or a snack while watching a game or a movie on TV. A substitute therefore has to be satisfying as well as healthy. Any manufactured snack product is likely to be as bad as chips, if not worse, so plan ahead and make your own.

5

Healthy alternatives

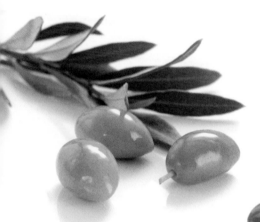

Become an olive connoisseur and enjoy the variety on offer.

Green olives
The ultimate "snack in a pack," green olives have a firm, crisp texture and a delicious, slightly astringent flavor that goes really well with chilled white wine. Choose a variety preserved in olive oil rather than brine and check the Ingredients List for "hidden" additives (see pages 64–65) such as MSG. A typical 1 oz (30 g) drained weight serving provides less than a third of the calories in chips, less than half the total fat, and only negligible saturated fat, carbohydrates, and sodium.

Eat seeds one by one so they take longer to eat—ideal for munching through films.

Kale chips
Low fat, low salt, low calorie, and so easy to make! Strip kale leaves from the tough stem, rinse and dry thoroughly, and rip pieces into a bowl. Spritz with olive oil and toss well, then scatter over a cookie sheet. Sprinkle lightly with unrefined sea salt and freshly ground black pepper, and bake in a preheated oven (350°F/180°C) until crisp (about 12 minutes), turning carefully once.

Tamari roasted seeds
Tamari is a more concentrated, less salty, and wheat-free version of soy sauce, with a rich, intensely savory taste. Toss pumpkin and sunflower seeds in a little tamari and roast on a cookie sheet in a preheated oven (300°F/150°C) for about 20 minutes, until crunchy. More filling than chips, and fiddly to eat, which effectively stops you being too greedy.

Dips
Part of the joy of eating chips is dunking them in a dip. Manufactured dips tend to be very salty, so whiz up your own in a blender, or even mash the ingredients together with a potato masher. Instead of chips, cut raw celery into sticks for dunking—it has a naturally salty flavor. Try:
• Hummus
• Guacamole
• Bean—fava, black, your favorite!

Tapas potatoes
Tapas potatoes will satisfy your flavor cravings. The potatoes are cut into chunks rather than thin slices, so there's far less surface area to absorb oil, and they're oven-baked rather than deep-fried. Mix a little unsalted tomato paste with a sprinkling of smoked paprika, a pinch of unrefined sea salt and a splash of olive oil, and toss 1-inch (2.5-cm) chunks of waxy potato in the mixture. Bake in a hot oven (400°F/200°C) until crisp and delicious. Enjoy!

Aging well

Aging is a natural and irreversible process. However, a healthy lifestyle, including being physically active and following a healthy diet, will help you enjoy your later years to the full.

Visit your dentist routinely. Adjust your dentures if they do not fit.

As you age, you may notice changes in your body shape, be less active, or be less interested in food. As we get older, we lose muscle—also called lean body mass—and get more fat mass. As a result, we need fewer calories. This has a negative impact on heart function and increases the risk of chronic diseases including heart disease (see pages 118–119), high blood pressure (see pages 116–117), and diabetes (see pages 114–115). Fat tends to concentrate in the trunk and it may increase the risk of hyperlipidemia (high levels of fat in your blood). During the aging process, we lose bone density for various reasons, including menopause in women. This can lead to osteoporosis or bone fractures.

Aging may also increase your needs for some nutrients. Iron and calcium intake sometimes are low. Moreover, vitamin B12 deficiency, which can result in pernicious anemia, is more common in the elderly. You may become more sensitive to dehydration because you may lose some of your sense of thirst and therefore not drink enough fluids.

Take heart, however, as it can be easy to adopt a few techniques and additions to your diet that will help you combat the main stresses and strains of the aging process.

> Eat an optimal diet and keep as active as you can—it's never too late to help your physical and mental health.

Dr. Joy Dauncey, Senior Scientist and Adviser in Nutritional and Biomedical Sciences, University of Cambridge, U.K.

Key food groups and how to attain them

	Benefits	Sources
Lutein and zinc	Can support hearing and vision during aging.	Lutein: Kale, turnip greens, and dandelion. Zinc: Sesame seeds, beans, and almonds.
Vitamin E	Antioxidant that can protect against the forming of free radicals in the body, which are dangerous to health.	Corn oil, soybean oil, margarine, and dressings.
Magnesium	Plays a role in preventing both stroke and heart attack. Increasing intake may decrease the risk of diabetes, asthma, and osteoporosis.	Spinach, fish, and beans.
Vitamin B12	Very important in blood synthesis; inadequate intake may cause anemia.	Low-fat dairy, fish, and lean red meat.
Vitamin B9/Folate	Important vitamin for making blood.	Beans, spinach, asparagus, and lentils.
Calcium and Vitamin D	Support bone health and help prevent osteoporosis.	Calcium: Dairy, especially low-fat milk, and artichokes. Vitamin D: Sun exposure, fish, fortified cereals, and dairy products.

Top 5 foods
HIGH IN VITAMIN B12

 Seafood
 Liver
 Dairy
 Fortified cereals
 Meat

 180

Food preparation

To make your food tender and easier to chew, cut it up, or chop, grind, or grate it, then steam or stew it. Unlike extensive boiling, this helps minimize loss of nutritional value. Soak dry beans before cooking, discard the soaking water, and place in fresh water to cook.

 179

Seven easy ways to increase calcium intake

1 Have two to four servings of dairy products every day—skim milk with cereal, yogurt as a midday snack, cheese sandwich at lunchtime, and chocolate milk in the evening.

2 To make sure you have some calcium at lunch, use low-fat cheese spread on your sandwich.

3 Sprinkle hard cheeses such as Parmesan or Romano on salads, meats, pasta, potatoes, cooked vegetables, eggs, and toast.

4 Use undiluted low-fat evaporated milk for soups or mashed potatoes instead of cream or butter.

5 Add powdered dry skim milk to your liquid skim milk for an additional boost of calcium and protein.

6 Make your oatmeal or hot cereal with low-fat milk instead of water.

7 If you are lactose intolerant, try lactose-free milk or calcium-fortified soymilk.

 181

Check these out

National Institute on Aging: www.nia.nih.gov/health/publication/healthy-eating-after-50
Healthy eating tips for the over-50s.
Nutrition.gov: www.nutrition.gov/life-stages/seniors
Nutrition advice for seniors.

 182

Seven easy ways to make sure you are drinking enough fluids

1 Drink plenty of water, milk, juice, and other fluids regularly to avoid dehydration, constipation, and kidney dysfunction. Drink at least five to eight glasses of fluids every day.

2 Take a tea "break" at least once per day.

3 Eat hearty vegetable soups for lunch.

4 Have cereal with low-fat milk for a snack instead of chips or sweets.

5 Drink fluids with each meal and snack and throughout the day.

6 Put 4 pints (2 L) of water in your refrigerator every day and make it a goal to drink it. Drink more if the weather is hot.

7 Keep a bottle of water at the front of the refrigerator shelf or an empty glass by the faucet. Have a glass of water every time you wash your hands.

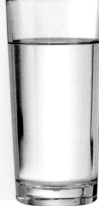

 Do this...

✓ Eat enough calories, even when eating alone.
✓ Keep your body fueled for the afternoon with a variety of whole-grain breads, lean protein, and fiber.
✓ Chop meats or hard foods so they are easier to chew.

 ...Not this

✗ Have an "easy" dinner of tea and toast that will not provide enough calories or nutrients.
✗ Skip meals: This causes your metabolism to slow down, which leads to you feeling sluggish and possibly making poorer choices later in the day.
✗ Avoid important food groups because the foods are too hard to chew.

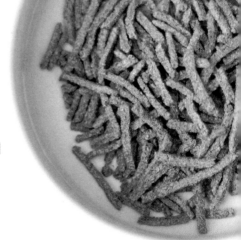

Nutrition for women

Just as your outlook on life changes over the years, so do your nutritional needs. Each life stage of womanhood brings new health challenges and opportunities.

Check out these facts to energize your body and stay healthy throughout the life cycle.

The teen years

With the transition through puberty comes an increased need for dietary iron. This is to offset the amount lost via monthly menstruation. In fact, the daily requirement for iron jumps from 8 to 15 milligrams (mg) at 14 years of age to meet the demand. See Top 5 sources of iron, below. Young women should build strong bones to help ward off osteoporosis later in life. Did you know that over 90% of adult bone mass has been formed by age 18? Three nutrients—calcium, phosphorus, and protein—make up most of the skeleton's weight: be sure to get enough of them throughout life.

Calcium: See 10 stellar sources, opposite.
Phosphorus: Fish, milk, yogurt, meat, cereal, nuts, and eggs.
Protein: Beans, meat, fish, milk, yogurt, soy milk, and nuts.

Pregnancy

Pregnancy presents many nutritional challenges as your body meets the baby's growth and nutritional demands.
Energy (calories): 300 additional calories each day.
Protein: 25 grams of extra protein per day, to total 71 grams a day.

Folate: Beans, orange juice, leafy green vegetables, black beans, fortified breakfast cereal, and grains.
Omega-3 fats: Salmon, tuna, mackerel, sardines, flaxseed oil, walnuts.
Choline: Eggs, milk, chicken, beef, pork, nuts.

Vitamin A: Liver, fish, milk, eggs, sweet potato, kale, broccoli, carrots.
Vitamin D: Salmon, sardines, mackerel, milk, fortified breakfast cereals.
Calcium: See 10 stellar sources, opposite.
Iron: See five top sources, below.
Fiber: 30 grams per day.

Motherhood and beyond

The years spent raising children and/or building a career are rewarding yet often stressful as well. Get in the habit of practicing excellent self-care: Caring for yourself first means you can better care for others.

• Eat meals and snacks that are regularly spaced throughout the day.
• Drink adequate fluid, particularly water, about 8 cups a day.
• Get plenty of sleep, typically 7–9 hours a night.

• Exercise daily, even if it's just a few five-minute walks.
• Reach out to others for emotional support.
• Look within by meditating for 10 minutes each day.

Top 5 sources of fiber, in grams per ½ cup		Top 5 sources of iron		Top 5 sources of protein	
Navy beans, cooked	9.5 g	Breakfast cereal, iron-fortified, 1 cup	8 mg	Milk, yogurt, 1 cup	8 g
Ready-to-eat bran cereal	8.8 g	Prune juice, ½ cup	4.5 mg	Fish, 1 oz (28 g)	7 g
Kidney beans, canned	8.2 g	Round steak, 3 oz (85 g)	3 mg	Meat, 1 oz (28 g)	7 g
Split peas, cooked	8.1 g	Baked beans, ½ cup	3 mg	Egg	7 g
Lentils, cooked	7.8 g	Spinach, cooked, ½ cup	2.3 mg	Beans, ½ cup	6.5 g

Hormonal imbalances

Many of the health issues women face are tied to unbalanced hormone levels. Learn more about these common conditions and you could soon feel good again.

Condition	Symptoms	Action
Perimenopause The gradual progression toward menopause. Many women start to notice changes in their forties, but it could happen earlier or later.	• Mood changes • Menstrual irregularity • Hot flashes, night sweats, sleep problems • Vaginal and bladder problems • Decreased estrogen levels—may contribute to unhealthy changes in cholesterol levels and to a loss of bone mass • Weight gain	• See your doctor if symptoms interfere with your wellbeing • Well-balanced, high-fiber diet, with emphasis on plant-based food for the natural phytoestrogens • Aerobic exercise and weight-bearing activities for strong bones • Adequate dietary calcium, vitamins D and K, and magnesium to protect bone health
Polycystic ovary syndrome (PCOS) Affects 5–10% of women of reproductive age; tends to run in families with history of infertility, menstrual problems, type 2 diabetes, or obesity.	• Menstrual irregularities • Overweightness or obesity • Abnormal facial and body hair • Insulin resistance • High testosterone levels • Infertility	• Weight loss of 5–10% of initial body weight • Individualized eating and exercise plan: whole grains, fruits, and vegetables high in antioxidants and fiber; regularly spaced meals; non-fat dairy products; marine sources of omega-3 fatty acids; carbohydrates with a low glycemic index • Medication
Hashimoto's disease Common cause of hypothyroidism, or low thyroid function; immune system attacks the thyroid gland, resulting in inflammation.	• Weight gain and fatigue • Constipation • Dry skin and puffy face • Increased sensitivity to cold • Muscle weakness and stiffness in joints	• Work with a registered dietitian to manage calories and weight; increase fruits, vegetables, and grains; limit saturated fats, if LDL levels (cholesterol) are too high • Supplemental thyroid hormone

Easy ways to treat your body to the nutrients it needs

By adding a little here and a little there, you can soon make sure your diet is maximizing on nutrients.

Sprinkle wheatgerm—a source of fiber and folic acid—on hot or dry cereal.

Make stews and soups in an iron pan to increase the iron content of foods.

Eat oatmeal for gut health and give yourself a facial with a paste of oatmeal, honey, and unflavored yogurt.

Make your own high-calcium and folic acid smoothie: Blend ice, milk, and orange juice or concentrate.

Use prune purée instead of sugar when making brownies or chocolate cakes, for added iron.

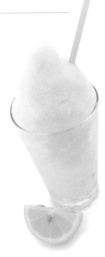

COUNTDOWN COUNTER

10 STELLAR SOURCES OF CALCIUM | MILLIGRAMS (MG) CALORIES

Beans, cooked, ½ cup | **60 mg**

Cottage cheese, low fat, ½ cup | **69 mg**

American cheese, 1 oz (30 g) | **175 mg**

Collard greens, cooked, ½ cup | **179 mg**

Pudding, milk-based, ½ cup | **185 mg**

Tofu, processed with calcium sulfate, 4 oz (110 g) | **200–420 mg**

Cheddar cheese, 1 oz (30 g) | **204 mg**

Skim milk, 1 cup | **301 mg**

Orange juice, with calcium, 1 cup | **350 mg**

Yogurt, low fat, 1 cup | **413 mg**

Nutrition for men

To be a healthy man is to achieve balance: a diet that provides enough, not excessive, calories; a lifestyle that allows for relaxation and exercise amid the stresses and strains of family and work demands.

Generally, men need more calories than women because they are typically bigger and have more muscle. The calorie needs for a man with a moderate physical activity is between 2,000 and 2,800 calories, but this depends on weight and height. However, men should be cautious about extra calories because abdominal fat has a direct correlation with the risk of heart disease—one of the major health risks for men, along with prostate cancer.

Drinking excessively may increase the risk of certain cancers—of the mouth, throat, esophagus, liver, and colon. High alcohol consumption may also interfere with testicular function and male hormone production, causing incapability and infertility. Excessive alcohol consumption may also contribute to abdominal obesity, which is a risk factor for diabetes mellitus, hypertension, and coronary heart disease.

But there is much you can do to remain in good health and shape.

Food groups for lifestyle

In men older than 30 years, being overweight, having a sedentary lifestyle, and an unhealthy diet are considered major causes of disease and death.

Men are typically meat eaters. Meat contains protein, iron, magnesium, zinc, vitamin E, and B vitamins, but may be high in saturated fat. Too much meat consumption may have a negative impact on heart health because of its fat content. For less fat, go with lean cuts.

Protein is necessary for exercise and building or rebuilding tissue but you can get it from many sources, not just meats. Protein foods include: lean meats, seafood, poultry, eggs, beans and peas, nuts, seeds, soy products, dairy products, and grains.

> Message for men planning to become dads: keeping fit and slim is great for you, and the physical and mental health of your future baby.

Dr. Joy Dauncey, Senior Scientist and Adviser in Nutritional and Biomedical Sciences, University of Cambridge, U.K.

Have a healthy lifestyle:

- Eat and drink healthily
- Be physically active
- Have regular checkups
- Get vaccinated
- Be smoke-free
- Prevent injuries
- Sleep well
- Manage stress

184 Packing in the nutrition

1 Make vegetables your main dish by topping a salad with your choice of a protein food.

2 Roast a whole chicken. When cooled, remove the skin, bones, and fat. Serve the meat as is, or use in a recipe.

3 Switch up your protein! Trade in your ham sandwich for one made with peanut butter, tuna, or canned salmon.

4 Vary your veggies by munching on cucumber, broccoli, or red and green peppers instead of chips when you have a sandwich at lunch.

5 Enjoy eggs as your protein food choice—up to one a day, on average, doesn't raise blood cholesterol levels. Top your salad with a hard-cooked egg to add protein and other nutrients.

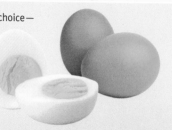

6 Pack a peanut butter and banana sandwich with a bag of homemade trail mix for lunch.

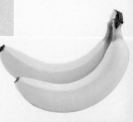

185
Use whole grains instead of refined grains

Whole grains are important sources of dietary fiber, B vitamins (thiamin, riboflavin, niacin, and folate), and minerals (iron, magnesium, and selenium). Consuming whole grains may reduce the risk of heart diseases and also some types of cancer.

186
Fishing for protein

Fish is a good source of protein, with low saturated fatty acids, and should be eaten two to three times per week. Some types of fish like salmon and herrings are good sources of omega-3 fatty acids that reduce the triglyceride level in the blood and also have an anti-inflammatory effect.

187
Apple pie protein shake
serves 1

This recipe contains a large serving of high-quality protein, important for repairing or building body tissues.

Ingredients

1 scoop vanilla whey protein
1 apple
1 cup vanilla Greek yogurt
Cinnamon
Water/Ice

Directions:
Blend all ingredients together to the desired consistency.

245 calories, 30 g protein

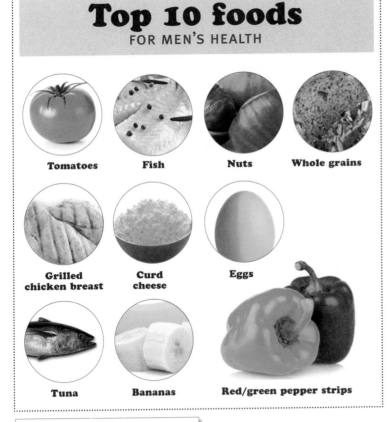

Top 10 foods
FOR MEN'S HEALTH

- Tomatoes
- Fish
- Nuts
- Whole grains
- Grilled chicken breast
- Curd cheese
- Eggs
- Tuna
- Bananas
- Red/green pepper strips

188
Cobb salad
serves 1

This recipe contains high-quality protein and vitamin B12 (turkey, egg) in addition to monounsaturated fats (avocado). The leafy greens provide some fiber, iron, niacin, and zinc.

Ingredients

2 oz (55 g) turkey, cubed
2 oz (55 g) avocado, cubed
1 egg, hard-cooked and chopped
1 cup fresh spinach

Directions:
Toss all the ingredients together and sprinkle with lemon juice or vinegar.

245 calories, 21 g protein

Do this...

✓ Be the best grill cook! When grilling or barbecuing, choose healthy options like veggie kabobs, grilled fish steaks, and low-calorie grilled chicken.

...Not this

✗ Fill your grill with hot dogs or fatty sausages and burgers.

189
Tomatoes for prostate

Eat tomatoes/tomato products at least once a week. Tomatoes are a good source of lycopene, which is an antioxidant that helps maintain a healthy prostate.

190
Stay in shape with fiber

Try to have at least 38 g of fiber every day and 30 g if you are 50 years or older. Consuming fiber may reduce the risk of heart diseases and constipation. When looking for best sources of fiber, check the Nutrition Facts label.
Excellent = 5 g or higher of fiber per serving
Good = 3 g or higher of fiber per serving

Nutrition for children

Habits are learned at a young age, so modeling healthy behaviors for children is important from the outset. However, as your child grows, so should their ability to make their own healthy decisions.

0–18 months

Infants: Breastfeeding

A baby will triple in weight and double in size in the first year. Breastmilk is filled with important carbohydrates, proteins, fats, vitamins, and minerals. Certain amino acids (building blocks of proteins) and fats, like DHA, are high in breastmilk and are an integral part of proper brain growth. The vitamins and minerals found in breastmilk are more bioavailable (better absorbed and used by the body) than those in formulas. The first few weeks of nursing can be difficult for mom and child, but if you are successful, it is the best nutrition you can offer your baby.

18 months– 4 years

Pre-schoolers: Playing and snacking

By throwing, spilling, and maybe eating their food, toddlers are learning about textures, amounts, distance, depth. How can you teach social and healthy eating habits at this age? With patience, a plan, and flexibility. A few of the important nutrients needed are calcium and vitamin D. After age two, offer low-fat cheeses and skim-to-low-fat milk as snack choices. Providing regularly timed, healthy snacks for pre-schoolers is important, enabling them to eat in short periods of time that are aligned with their appetite and attention span.

4–10 years

School age: Off to a good start

Breakfast is the most important meal of the day, especially for children. This will provide the necessary nutrients to help them power through their school day. Make a breakfast with a high-quality protein like eggs and add a piece of whole-wheat bread toasted with just a dab of jam. Also, provide nutritious after-school snacks that will get them through until dinner, such as graham crackers with peanut butter. Help your school-age child to make healthier choices by being physically active. After all the homework is done, encourage sports with friends and active play.

11–13 years

Tweens: Convenience for on the go

Tweens are likely grabbing the most convenient choices that are high in calories. Pack a low-fat yogurt for their day. Encourage them to drink low-fat or skim milk or water. They are always on the go, but don't let your tween stand while eating. Encourage dinnertime to be a time when the family sits together and talks about their day.

14–18 years

Teens: Responsible power snacking

These individuals want to make their own decisions, so talk to your teen about healthy choices and physical activity. Popular sugary, caffeinated drinks are empty calories so encourage power snacks and drinks like low-fat milk and homemade fruit smoothies. Watch for disordered eating at this age. If you think your child is not eating enough, skipping meals or whole food groups, then talk with him or her, and if warranted, contact a health-care professional.

(191) Five things you may be doing to sabotage your kids' eating habits

1 Making a face when you see certain foods (vegetables or fruits) put on your own plate.

2 Ordering soda instead of water in front of your kids.

3 Eating while standing up at the kitchen table.

4 Encouraging your child to finish their plate. Forcing a child to eat when not hungry or once full predisposes the child to overeating.

5 Creating a sweets-based reward system and unhealthy food chain by encouraging your child to eat a good dinner so that they can have dessert.

192 Get moving

Increasing physical activity and reducing sedentary behavior are just as important as proper nutrition for a growing child. Get up off the couch and try out some of these ideas with your children:
• Put on some fun music and dance around the house.
• Go for a long bike ride and talk about your day and the beautiful surroundings at dinnertime.
• Go window-shopping with your teenage daughter for a good walk.

Never offer a sweet or unhealthy treat as a reward for good behavior or for doing chores. Offer praise and your time and attention instead.

Five easy snacks

1 Fresh fruit

2 Homemade trail mix (nuts, dried fruit, whole-wheat cereal)

3 Peanut butter spread on celery

4 Leftovers

5 Whole-grain cereal with skim milk

193 Picky eater strategies

Involve your child in the food prep and give them options.

Praise all attempts at trying new foods.

Let them dip fun finger foods such as carrot sticks in low-fat ranch dressing or homemade hummus.

Add some diced or blended veggies into their favorite dish.

Involve your child in the food-preparation process.

 Do this...

✓ Enjoy physical activity with your kids.
✓ Talk about the good things your kids did that day during the family meal.
✓ Have a range of healthy meal enders such as fruit salad or herbal tea.
✓ Have a favorite healthy food day per family member, such as Dad's Friday, Mom's Monday, Toddler Tom's Tuesday, Tween Kimberly's Thursday.
✓ Try a different preparation method for a food if it is not liked the first time it is served.

 ...Not this

✗ Make exercise a chore or something they have to do.
✗ Argue with or reprimand your children at the dinner table.
✗ Always have a cake or sweet after a meal.
✗ Make all meals based on just one family member's preferences.
✗ Give up and never try serving the food again. Sometimes you just have to find a preparation method that is liked!

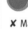

194 Follow these guidelines for a heart-healthy diet

1 Have them select the dinner vegetable. Give parameters such as "a green one," etc.

2 Have them select where the family will eat out. Give parameters such as "price range, must include salad options," etc.

3 Make sure the television is off and the whole family is sitting down for dinner.

4 Have them take one bite of their food and tell the family what their favorite part of the food is, whether it's flavor, texture, taste, etc.

5 Make a healthy dessert together like low-fat frozen yogurt with a small dab of their favorite topping.

Fueling the athlete

The diets of highly active people require more fluid and energy, and are a crucial component of athletic success.

For the average exerciser (someone who participates in moderate intensity fitness for 60 minutes or less, one to five days a week), specific nutrition strategies are not really necessary to ensure optimal performance. However, if you typically train for a minimum of 60 minutes, five to seven days a week, your nutrition (and rest) is just as important as your training sessions.

Before training or competition
In order to perform your best, your body needs fuel in your system. Consuming a meal or snack and adequate fluids between 60 minutes and 4 hours prior to training is ideal for providing this necessary fuel. Choose foods that are familiar to you, high in carbohydrate content, moderate in protein, and low in fat. The quantity of food should decrease the closer you are eating to the start time of your training session. Experiment with different meal and snack options until you find one that digests easily and makes you feel energized.

During training or competition
Carbohydrate intake during training or competition has been shown to effectively extend athletic performance. In endurance sports (distance running, cycling, swimming, or the like) as well as prolonged practices lasting at least 60 minutes, taking in at least 60–90 g of carbohydrate per hour is recommended. It is best to spread this intake out over the training period, ingesting about 30 g of carbohydrate every 15–20 minutes from the start.

After training or competition
The need for a post-training meal is dependent on the intensity and duration of the workout, as well as when the next high-intensity workout will occur. Intense workouts lasting longer than 90 minutes should be followed by a carbohydrate-rich meal containing high-glycemic-index foods to help replenish muscle glycogen stores. This is especially important if you plan to have more than one workout a day or have strenuous workouts on back-to-back days. Adding about 20–25 g of protein to your post-training meal has been found to support muscle repair and building, and is important for both strength and endurance athletes.

Hydration
Athletes require more fluid due to greater sweat loss. To prepare for training or competition, athletes should drink about 1–3 cups (250–750 ml), depending on body size, in the 4 hours prior to the event. During training, drink water, about 2–4 sips every 15 minutes, and use sports beverages to provide energy and replenish electrolytes if you are working for more than an hour. It is especially important if you are a heavy or salty sweater to closely monitor sweat loss and be diligent about replacing lost fluids. To do this, weigh yourself before and after training or competition. For each pound of body weight lost, drink 16–24 fl oz (475–700 ml) of fluid in the time immediately following the completion of training.

> Pay attention to combinations of power foods that work particularly well for helping you feel fueled and energized for your workouts. These are unique to each person and may be something off the beaten path of your regular food choices.
>
> Jenna Braddock, Consultant and Sports Dietitian, University of North Florida

- **Fuel early and often for optimal performance during endurance sports.**
- **Nutrition, hydration, and rest are just as important as training.**
- **Carbs are fuel for your body. Protein is the building blocks. Both are important.**

 Do this...

✓ To perform at your best, always have some sort of fuel in your system before working out.

✓ Choose moderate-protein pre-workout foods like granola bars, a lean-meat sandwich, peanut butter and jelly sandwich, or low-fat yogurt.

✓ Practice different food options before, during, and after exercise to find the combination that works for your body, and have a plan for training and competition.

 ...Not this

✗ Fast or eat a heavy-fat meal in the hours prior to an event.

✗ Have extremely high-protein shakes (more than 40 g protein).

✗ Try something new or rely on event planners for your nutrition before an event.

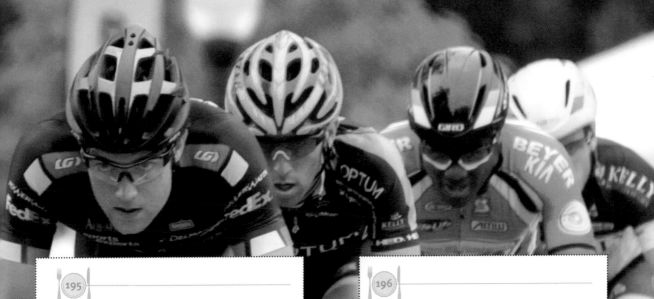

PRE-EVENT NUTRITION

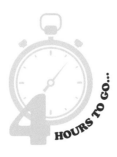

Eat a full meal including high carbohydrate, moderate protein, and low fat
Example: Sub sandwich on whole-grain bread with turkey, cheese, and vegetables and a piece of fruit.
+ 1–3 cups (250–750 ml) of water, depending on body size, in the 4 hours prior to the event.

4 HOURS TO GO...

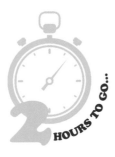

Eat a large snack consisting mostly of carbohydrate
Example: Low-fat yogurt and banana.

2 HOURS TO GO...

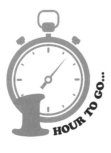

Eat a small snack that you are familiar with and is almost completely simple carbohydrate
Example: Sports gel or bar; piece of fruit.

1 HOUR TO GO...

EVENT NUTRITION

Consume foods with 15 g of carbohydrate every 15–20 minutes during exercise or competition lasting longer than 1 hour:
- 8 fl oz (230 ml) of a sports drink
- 15 jellybeans
- 1 mini peppermint patty candy
- About 3–4 orange slices
- One small banana
- ½ sachet of energy gel
- ¼ energy bar (varies by brand)

+ 2–4 sips of water every 15 minutes

POST-EVENT NUTRITION

Replenish with a carbohydrate-rich meal containing high-glycemic-index foods, such as:
- Large baked sweet potato
- Corn and black bean salad
- Large roll

Add a grilled chicken breast for protein.

+ For each pound of body weight lost, drink 16–24 fl oz (475–700 ml) of water immediately following the completion of training.

Food and mood

Do the foods you eat affect your mood and productivity? Research says they do, and you can change how you feel by following a few simple steps.

A cup of coffee may give a morning boost, but too much will give you jitters. Check your tolerance levels.

Are you alert and invigorated in the morning, grouchy before lunch, or cranky mid-afternoon, or does your mood improve as the day goes on? Some of us are naturally morning people and others come to life in the afternoon or evening. If you want to change your mood, what should you change about your food?

Brain science

The neurochemicals in the brain most associated with mood are serotonin, dopamine, norepinephrine, and melatonin. While certain nutrients are needed for the production of these brain chemicals, their regulation may be more a function of particular foods than individual nutrients unless you have a deficiency.

While individual nutrients do not correct mental health problems, if you are low in them, adding more can make a difference to how you feel. You want your brain to be at optimal performance for maximum cognitive ability, so eating well is important.

The bottom line is that what you eat and drink can influence your brain chemistry, which then affects your mood. Awareness of your particular patterns of intake and mood changes can be gained by keeping a food and mood record for a week or so. Writing down everything you eat and drink for that length of time will give you clues about the particular relationship between food eaten regularly or sporadically, and associated changes in mood.

Eat breakfast!

Avoid the midmorning slump.

199

Check your caffeine intake

Caffeine has been shown to increase alertness, productivity, and even athletic performance—but it has also been linked to irritability, anxiety, and mood swings. Different people have different tolerance levels: some cannot sleep at night if they consume caffeine in the afternoon; others enjoy an espresso before bed. Get to know your own reactions to the stimulant and assess whether your intake suits them. If you decide to reduce or eliminate caffeine consumption, do so gradually, to prevent the withdrawal symptoms of headaches and body aches. Be aware, too, that energy drinks and other soft drinks can be loaded with caffeine.

198 Mood-enhancing guidelines

1 Eat Mediterranean style. In a recent study, foods typical of the Mediterranean style of eating were associated with positive effects (good mood) while Western diet foods were associated with low positive effects and negative emotions in women. Mediterranean foods in the study were fresh vegetables, fresh fruits, milk, cheese, olive oil, nuts, fish, and legumes. Western foods in the study were red meat, processed meats, fast food, sweets and desserts, and soft drinks or soda.

2 Have a snack, especially if you only ate a light meal. Snacking has been associated with improved mood. See pages 34–35 for some healthy snack ideas.

3 Combine protein and a carbohydrate for increased alertness. Eating a carbohydrate alone as a snack can cause a blood sugar increase followed by a decrease that can negatively influence concentration and mood. Protein contributes to satiety, making you feel more satisfied.

For some, cookies are a snack comfort food. If you must indulge, make it a small, single cookie and favor one with oatmeal or nuts.

Do this...

✓ Use mealtimes to talk about positive events of the day or good news. This will create positive associations with food.

...Not this

✗ Quarrel, reprimand, or discuss bad news. Avoid associating food with negative feelings.

200

Comfort eating

Tempted to overeat when you are angry or sad? Plan and avoid the associated weight gain by eating low-calorie foods (avoid sweets and high-salt and fat foods) and increasing physical activity to boost energy and mood. If you are feeling grouchy, reflect and determine if maybe you are just hungry. If so, pick up a yogurt, a piece of low-fat cheese and fruit, a glass of milk, and a few nuts.

201

The chocolate debate

Some recent studies have pointed toward cognitive enhancement following ingestion of chocolate; other studies have not. In most cases, alterations in brain activation patterns following chocolate consumption have been determined. However, it is unclear whether the effects of chocolate on the brain are due to the sensory effects of eating chocolate or pharmacological actions of the chocolate constituents like cocoa flavanols or methylxanthines. More research is needed; in the meantime, a little of what you fancy may well do you some good.

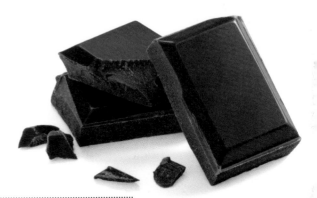

The science of whether, physiologically, chocolate affects mood is still unclear— but enjoying a small piece of dark chocolate will surely make you smile!

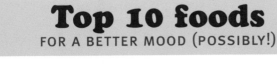

Top 10 foods
FOR A BETTER MOOD (POSSIBLY!)

Fresh vegetables

Fresh fruit

Milk

Cheese

Olive oil

Nuts

Fish

Legumes

Dark chocolate

Water

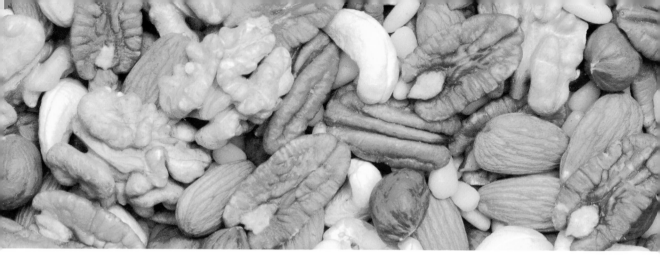

Food allergies

Food allergies can be serious, even life-threatening, conditions.
By learning more about the diagnosis and treatment of an allergy,
you'll be on your way to vibrant health.

Have you experienced bloating, flatulence, hives, nasal congestion, diarrhea, or an itchy dermatitis after eating a particular food? Could a food allergy be the cause of your symptoms? It's possible. If you have one, however, you don't have to face a lifetime of tummy troubles and bland eating. Armed with an accurate diagnosis and a hefty dose of nutrition education, you can learn to manage your food allergy and will soon feel good again.

Diagnosis

Over 90% of all food allergies are due to eight foods: wheat, milk, eggs, soy, peanuts, tree nuts, fish, and shellfish. Whatever the offending food, it's critical that an accurate diagnosis is obtained. Technically, a food allergy— also called food hypersensitivity— occurs when the immune system reacts to a food protein that the body mistakenly identifies as harmful. The reaction can occur almost instantly or within 2 hours of ingesting, inhaling, or coming into contact with the food. In contrast, intolerance is an adverse reaction to a food caused by other

> **Prevalence of food allergy has almost doubled during the past 20 years.**
>
> Jackie Shank, Didactic Program in Dietetics Director and Nutrition Instructor, University of North Florida

means. For instance, the following can cause symptoms in susceptible people:
• **Phenylethylamine** A substance in aged cheese, chocolate, and red wine
• **Sulfites** In dried fruits and vegetables, wine, and beer
• **Tartrazine** A yellow food dye in many orange- and yellow-colored processed foods

An accurate clinical history will help your doctor make the correct diagnosis, so be prepared to answer a lot of questions about your symptoms and the suspected foods. Additional diagnostic tools include:
• Keeping a detailed food and symptom diary

• A physical examination to look for skin abnormalities and signs of poor nutrition
• Laboratory tests such as the skin prick test (or SPT—a common, simple, safe, and fast allergy test in which a minute amount of allergen is "pricked" into the skin to check for a small localized response such as a bump or redness) and two blood tests: the radioallergosorbent test (RAST), and the enzyme-linked immunosorbent assay (ELISA)
• An elimination diet.

Easy substitutions	
Instead of...	...Try this
Store-bought trail mix	Homemade sulfite-free trail mix
Wheat flour	Rice, millet, quinoa, corn, lentils
Cows' milk	Rice milk
Egg (in baking)	1 tablespoon ground flaxseed mixed with 3 tablespoons lukewarm water

 Do this...   **...Not this**

✓ See a qualified medical professional for an accurate diagnosis if you suspect that you or your child may have one or more food allergies. This same professional can guide you through an elimination diet and food challenge (see below).

✗ Try to diagnose yourself and start omitting food groups from your diet.

 (202)

Eating away from home

If you're unsure about the establishment, why take a chance? Bring safe food with you. Ask detailed questions about menu items and their preparation. If you use medicine, be sure to carry it with you at all times.

 (203)

Elimination diet

You'll eliminate all forms of the possible offending foods (for example, wheat, eggs, milk, nuts, fish, shellfish, and soy). Then you add each one back slowly, over time, while carefully noting your symptoms. You may have to repeat the test to confirm the allergy. Nutritional supplements might be needed if multiple foods are removed from the diet for longer than 14 days.

After your symptoms have completely resolved and you're feeling much better, a food challenge is conducted, during which you'll be checked for the recurrence of symptoms after consumption of the suspected food allergen. This should only be done in a medical setting to ensure your safety.

Label reading and grocery shopping

Food manufacturers are continually updating their products so be sure to check nutrition labels often. Both the U.S. and the U.K. have regulations that require the disclosure of the most common food allergens in the product's ingredient list. You can often find additional information on company websites or by emailing a customer service representative.

 (204)

Check these out

Food Allergy Research and Education (FARE): www.foodallergy.org
Extensive information about allergies; tools and resources for managing them in all aspects of life.

American Academy of Allergy, Asthma, and Immunology (AAAAI): www.aaaai.org
Authoritative, expert resources to make informed decisions regarding allergies, asthma, and immune deficiency disorders.

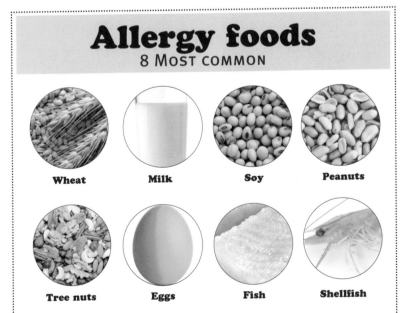

Allergy foods
8 MOST COMMON

Wheat   Milk   Soy   Peanuts

Tree nuts   Eggs   Fish   Shellfish

Gluten sensitivity

It is important to establish if you have celiac disease or a sensitivity to gluten, so if you suspect one or the other, make sure you get tested by a qualified health professional so you do not subject yourself to unnecessary food restrictions.

Celiac disease is an immune reaction to foods containing gluten that results in breakdown of the intestines. Many people who think they have celiac disease may actually have sensitivity to gluten—a less-severe reaction to foods containing gluten that does not damage the intestines—and it may be more common than celiac disease.

Gluten is a protein in wheat, barley, and rye. People with gluten sensitivity may have the same type of reaction when they eat foods with gluten as people with celiac disease, such as diarrhea, abdominal pain, and bloating. Symptoms of gluten sensitivity may also include headache, joint pain, and a numb feeling in the arms, legs, or fingers.

There is no diagnostic test that can tell you if you have gluten sensitivity.

If you have symptoms after eating foods containing gluten, see a physician to test for celiac disease. If negative, your physician may recommend you stop eating foods with gluten. If your symptoms go away, you may have gluten sensitivity.

Adapting to the diagnosis

If you are diagnosed with gluten sensitivity, you should be able to reduce or eliminate your symptoms with a gluten-free diet (see below).

Living gluten free takes time, as you learn how to change your diet. Once you work through the changes, it will become much easier. You will find that it is well worth the effort when you are free from the symptoms of gluten sensitivity.

Liven up your gluten-free meal by trying:
Amaranth bread
Buckwheat (kasha) pancakes
Cornmeal porridge (polenta)
Millet muffins
Oatmeal bread
Potato (baked or boiled)
Quinoa and beans
Brown rice pilaf
Sweet potato (baked or boiled)
Wild rice casserole

Gluten free and with high nutritional value, sweet potatoes are a healthy option, despite containing more sugar than white potatoes.

Gluten-free pasta substitutes include:
- **Barley**
- **Rice (including wild rice)**
- **Potatoes**
- **Ethnic root vegetables: water chestnuts, green plantains, cassava**

 205 | **Gluten-free diet**

1 A gluten-free diet can be high in calories and low in fiber, iron, calcium, and vitamins A, D, E, K, and the B vitamins.

2 Focus your meals on fruit, vegetables, protein, dairy foods, and gluten-free grains. You can use flours made from beans, peas, or seeds to replace wheat flour.

3 Distillation removes gluten, so choose distilled alcohol or wine instead of beer or drinks with mixers. You can also use distilled vinegars.

4 There are gluten-free products available; just be sure to choose foods that fit in with your overall diet goals and are not high in extra calories or sugar.

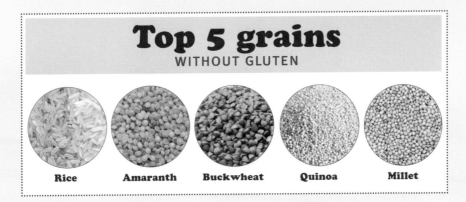

Top 5 grains
WITHOUT GLUTEN

Rice   **Amaranth**   **Buckwheat**   **Quinoa**   **Millet**

 206

Foods to avoid

To eat gluten free, avoid foods that naturally contain gluten, such as wheat, barley, and rye as well as bran, bulgur, couscous, durum/semolina flour (pasta), orzo, whole-wheatberries, spelt, farina, kasha, beer, and matzoh.

Other foods may also have gluten from processing or additives. You must read Ingredients Lists on food packages for hidden sources of gluten. These foods include oats, luncheon meats, energy bars, candy, baked beans, nuts, ice cream, soups, salad dressings, soy sauce, vinegars, marinades, flavorings, seasonings, some alcohol, vitamins, and supplements.

 207

Check these out

www.celiaccentral.org/non-celiac-gluten-sensitivity
Basic information about non-celiac gluten sensitivity.
www.ext.colostate.edu/pubs/foodnut/09375.html
Gluten-free diet guide for people newly diagnosed with celiac disease, including lists of foods to include/avoid and a long list of resources.
www.ext.colostate.edu/pubs/foodnut/09376.html
Gluten-free baking guide including flour substitutions for types of baked goods.
www.celiaccentral.org/gluten-free-recipes
Easy gluten-free recipes from the National Foundation for Celiac Awareness.

 208   **Raspberry ice**   serves **1**

This gluten-free sweet dish provides antioxidants, fiber, vitamins, and minerals while increasing your fruit intake.

Ingredients

1 cup frozen raspberries

Syrup (¼ cup water with 2 tbsp sugar)

Directions:
Purée frozen raspberries with a small amount of syrup to the desired consistency and sweetness. Serve immediately or store in the freezer and let thaw slightly before serving.

162 calories

 Do this...

✓ Make some healthy whole-grain side dishes that provide carbohydrates to help you with satiety and a feeling of fullness.

 ...Not this

✗ Make a lot of fried potatoes or other fried foods to help you feel full. They are loaded with calories and fat.

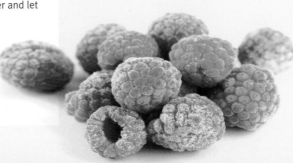

Glossary

Aerobic fitness An individual's ability to exercise for a long period of time without getting out of breath. Also referred to as *cardiovascular fitness*. Both terms refer to how efficiently an individual transports oxygen that is breathed into the body, through the cardiovascular system into the exercising muscle cells, where it can help to make energy, allowing physical movement to continue.

Alcohol (Also known as *ethanol* or *grain alcohol*) An intoxicating beverage made from fermented sugars. Beverages such as wine, beer, whiskey, gin, and vodka contain alcohol, which provides 7 calories per gram.

Blanche Immerse in boiling water for a very short period of time. This helps with vegetable or fruit skin removal, and to slow ripening and enzymatic action. Often done prior to other preparation or freezing.

Calorie The measure of energy a certain food provides. In scientific terms, a calorie is the amount of energy needed to raise the temperature of one gram of water by one degree Celsius. When referring to food, the measure is a *kilocalorie*, which is the energy needed to raise the temperature of one kilogram of water by one degree Celsius. This measure (*kcalories*) is used in the United States to measure the energy in foods, but in other parts of the world the measure used may be the *joule*.

Calorie dense Foods that are high in calories and low in nutrients, commonly called *junk* or *empty-calorie foods*. (See *nutrient dense*.)

Carbohydrate Compounds made of single (simple) sugars or multiple (complex) compounds that may be in the form of digestible starches or nondigestible fibers such as celluloses. Digestible carbohydrates such as starches and sugars provide 4 calories per gram.

Chronic disease Thought to be mostly caused by lifestyle and environmental causes, chronic diseases take time, even decades, to develop, and often do not have initial symptoms. Examples include heart disease, stroke, obesity, and some types of cancers.

Electrolytes Electrically charged ions that dissolve in water and are important in the body's fluid balance both within and outside the cells.

Energy The capacity to do work. Energy from food is measured in and referred to as calories, and is absorbed during digestion.

Fats Consist of a large group of compounds, known as *lipids* that are either solid (fats) or liquid (oils) at room temperature. Fats play a role in body temperature regulation, cell function, and organ insulation. Eating too many solid fats can lead to cardiovascular disease, while eating liquid oils has protective qualities. Recommended intake is approximately 30 percent of total calories, based on adequate caloric intake for healthy weight maintenance.

Fiber, dietary The non-starchy parts of plant foods that are not digested. There are two types important for colon health—soluble and non-soluble. Soluble fiber dissolves in water and is associated with lowering cholesterol; non-soluble does not dissolve and helps promote regularity of bowel movements.

Flexibility The extent to which an individual is able to move body joints through complete range of motion. Can be improved by engaging in specific forms of exercise such as stretching and yoga.

Food exchange system Diet-planning tools that group foods according to their nutrient content and/or calories. Ensures that the same calories or grams of carbohydrates are being consumed.

Glucose A carbohydrate that is a simple sugar; the body's main source of energy, used in metabolism. Glucose is essential, and the only form of energy used by the nervous system and red blood cells.

Glycemic Index (GI) Ranks foods with carbohydrates on a scale from 0 to 100 according to how much they raise blood sugar levels after eating compared to a reference amount of sugar or white bread.

Glycogen Glucose stored in the liver and muscles, used when blood glucose levels are low or during exercise.

Grazing Eating several (five or more) small meals or snacks throughout the day.

High blood pressure The force of blood pushing against the walls of the arteries as the heart pumps blood. Consistently high blood pressure may damage important organs of the body such as the heart and/or kidneys.

High-density lipoprotein (HDL) Found in blood and a component of total cholesterol. Considered the "good cholesterol," levels of about 60 mg/dL or higher have been shown to be protective against heart disease.

Hydrogenation In relation to food, the process of adding hydrogen to a liquid fat to make it solid. The trans fats created as part of this process are associated with increased risk for heart disease.

Insulin resistance Cellular resistance to the sugar-regulating hormone insulin; results in an undesirable increase of blood glucose levels.

Lactose Naturally found sugar in milk; digested with the help of the enzyme lactase, which breaks down lactose into two simple sugars called glucose and galactose. If a person does not produce enough or any lactase, he or she may have difficulty digesting unfermented milk products. Among the symptoms are bloating and gas, and mild to severe nausea, cramps, and diarrhea.

Symptom severity depends on the amount of lactose tolerated, digestion rate, meal combination, etc. Lactose intolerance is sometimes confused with milk allergy, which is an immune-system reaction to the proteins, not the sugars, in milk.

Low-density lipoprotein (LDL) Component of total cholesterol. Considered the "bad cholesterol," levels of above 100 mg/dL have been shown to be a major risk factor for developing heart disease.

Metabolic syndrome A combination of insulin resistance or high fasting blood sugar, abdominal obesity, high blood pressure, low HDL cholesterol, and high blood triglycerides that increase a person's risk of cardiovascular disease.

Mindful eating An awareness and focused emphasis on experiencing the present moment and activity, in order to make more appropriate self-care and food choices.

Minerals Inorganic non-calorie (energy) elements found in varying amounts and forms in human bodies and in the earth. Minerals required in human nutrition have a specific role or function in the body. In nutrition, the major minerals include calcium, phosphorus, sodium, potassium, magnesium, chloride, and sulfate.

Monounsaturated fats Have one unsaturated fatty acid in their chemical compound; from plant sources and are liquid at room temperature. This type of fat may help raise the "good" HDL cholesterol and is considered an ideal source of dietary fat.

Muscular endurance The ability to do repeated muscular work or contractions against some kind of resistance over an extended time period.

Muscular strength The maximum amount of force that a muscle group can exert while working against some kind of resistance or object of some sort, such as a weight.

Nutrient dense or nutrient rich Food that is high in one or more nutrients relative to the amount of calories it contains; that is, the ratio of nutrients to the total energy (calorie) content is high. Nutrient-dense foods provide a large amount of vitamins and minerals with few calories. (See *calorie dense*.)

Nutrigenomics Integration of genetics and other sciences to human nutrition. A new discipline that is expected to affect future nutrition care because differences in genotype should impact the relationship between diet and health at individual levels.

Omega-3 and omega-6 fats Polyunsaturated fats (PUFAs) with a variety of functions in the human body. Plant sources such as soybeans and sunflower seeds are sources of vegetable oils that contain omega-6 fats. Certain nuts (almonds and walnuts) and seafood, especially fatty fish (tuna and salmon), are good sources of omega-3 fats, which are known for contributing to heart and brain health and for reducing inflammation.

Phytonutrients or phytochemicals Compounds or chemicals found in plants that are not required in a diet, but have been found to be beneficial to health.

Plant stanols or sterols Similar to cholesterol but found in plants. Help remove "bad" cholesterol from the body.

Polyunsaturated fats Derive their name from their chemical structure, because there is more than one site of unsaturated fatty acids. These fats are liquid at room temperature and may help reduce total cholesterol.

Portion The amount of food selected to be eaten at a meal or snack by an individual. Not to be confused with a *serving size* (see below). Portions chosen by the general population have increased over time, such that "larger" sizes have become the norm. This is known as *portion distortion*.

Protein Compounds made up of multiple arrangements of amino acids. Some amino acids are not made by the body and must be obtained through foods (essential amino acids). Proteins provide 4 calories per gram.

Safe foods Prepared hygienically and sourced responsibly; not from a food safety recall or illness outbreak. For persons who have food allergies, a safe food is free from ingredients that may provoke a reaction.

Serving size The recommended amount of food to be served. This differs from a *portion* (see above).

Sugar alcohols Types of sweetener, which do not actually contain alcohol, but do include erythritol, glycerol, isomalt, lactitol, maltitol, mannitol, sorbitol, and xylitol. While considered safe, some people may experience stomach trouble as a result of consuming too much at one time.

Trans fats Mostly occur as a result of creating a solid fat from liquid oil through the process of partial or full hydrogenation of plant oils. Also occur naturally in some meat and dairy products but in small quantities. Consumption of trans fats, which are most common in foods processed with hydrogenated fats, has been associated with increased risk of heart disease.

Vitamins Non-caloric compounds of nutrients that are required in very small amounts and are essential for metabolism. Deficiency of these compounds may be harmful. Vitamins are divided into two groups: fat soluble and water soluble. Fat-soluble vitamins include A, D, E, and K; water-soluble vitamins include B and C.

Resources

At home
- www.styleathome.com
- www.stilltasty.com
- www.thekitchn.com

Calorie information
- http://caloriecount.about.com
- www.fatsecret.com
- www.fitday.com/webfit/nutrition
- www.livestrong.com
- http://ndb.nal.usda.gov/ndb
- http://nutritiondata.self.com
- www.sparkpeople.com

Cooking
- American Association of Family and Consumer Sciences. 2001. *Food: A Handbook of Terminology, Purchasing, & Preparation.* American Association of Family and Consumer Sciences
- Bennion, M., Scheule, B. 2000. *Introductory Foods.* Prentice Hall
- Herbst ST, Herbst R. (2007) *The New Food Lover's Companion.* Barron's Educational Series
- www.bhg.com/recipes
- www.cdkitchen.com
- www.cookinglight.com
- www.ehow.com
- http://everydaylife.globalpost.com/blanch-red-potatoes-peeling-31680.html
- www.finecooking.com/recipes
- www.gardenersnet.com/recipes
- www.healwithfood.org/chart/vegetable-steaming-times.php
- www.livestrong.com
- http://recipes.howstuffworks.com
- http://thaifood.about.com
- www.vegancoach.com

Cultural foods
- Kittler, PG, Sucher, KP. (2008) *Food and Culture.* Thomson Wadsworth
- Zibat, E. (2010) *The Ethnic Food Lover's Companion: A Sourcebook for Understanding the Cuisines of the World.* Menasha Ridge Press
- www.delish.com/recipes/cooking-recipes/healthy-soul-food-0pro910
- www.eatingwell.com/recipes_menus/recipe_slideshows/soul_food_recipes
- www.foodbycountry.com/Spain-to-Zimbabwe-Cumulative-Index/Spain.html
- www.jnto.go.jp/eng/attractions/dining/food/jfood_01.html
- www.nrdc.org/health/effects/mercury/sushi.asp
- www.pbs.org/independentlens/soul-food-junkies/recipes.html
- www.rd.com/health/healthy-eating/healthy-eating-best-bets-for-chinese-takeout
- www.webmd.com/diet/features/diets-of-world-japanese-diet

Diets
- Agatston, A. (2011) *The South Beach Diet.* Rodale
- American Dietetic Association. (2009) Position of the American Dietetic Association: Vegetarian Diets. *Journal of the American Dietetic Association.* 109(107): 1266–1282
- Amsden, M. (2013) *The RAWvolution Continues: The Living Foods Movement in 150 Natural and Delicious Recipes.* Simon & Schuster, Inc., Atria Books
- Bolduan, J. (2011) *Green Smoothie Detox Diet.* WP Enterprise, Inc.
- Carmody, RN, Wrangham, RW (2009) The Energetic Significance of Cooking. *Journal of Human Evolution.* 57:379–291
- Cordain, L. (2010) *The Paleo Diet.* Houghton Mifflin Harcourt
- Craig, W.J. (2010) Nutrition Concerns and Health Effects of Vegetarian Diets. *Nutrition in Clinical Practice.* 25:613
- Cruise, J. (2006) *The 3-Hour Diet.* HarperCollins Publishers
- D'Adamo, P, Whitney, C. (1997) *Eat Right for Your Type.* Putnam
- Diamond, H., Diamond, M. (2010) *Fit for Life.* Grand Central Life & Style
- Dukan, P. (2011) *Dukan Diet.* Crown Publishing Group Random House
- Ellerbeck, Susan. (2014) *The Raw Food Diet for Beginners.* CreateSpace Independent Publishing Platform
- Guiliano, Mireille. (2013) *French Women Don't Get Fat.* William Morrow
- Link, LB, Jacobson, JS (2008) Factors Affecting Adherence to a Raw Vegan Diet. *Complementary Therapies in Clinical Practice.* 14:53-59
- Marcus, E. *The Ultimate Vegan Guide: Compassionate Living without Sacrifice.* 2011
- Mitchell, S, Christie, C. *Fat is Not Your Fate: Outsmart Your Genes and Lose the Weight Forever.* Simon & Schuster. 2005
- Mullin, GE (2010) Popular Diets Prescribed by Alternative Practitioners—Part 2. *Nutrition in Clinical Practice.* 25:308
- Niemerow, A. (2012). *Super Cleanse.* William Morrow
- Perricone, N. (2010) *Forever Young.* Simon & Schuster, Inc., Atria Books
- Harrison, K. (2013) *5-2 Diet.* Ulysses Press
- Rodriguez, JC. (Ed.). (2007) *The Diet Selector.* Running Press
- Rolls, B. (2011) *Volumetrics.* Harper Collins
- Tribole, E, Resch, E. (2012) *Intuitive Eating.* St. Martin's Griffin
- Westman, Eric C, Phinney, Stephen D. and Volek, Jeff S. (2010) *The New Atkins for a New You: The Ultimate Diet for Shedding Weight and Feeling Great.* Fireside
- www.bing.com/videos/search?q=Ted+Paleo+diet
- www.nwcr.ws/Research

- http://weirdworldofhumans.wordpress.com/2009/06
- http://ybefit.byu.edu/Portals/88/Documents/How%20Does%20The%20BOD%20POD%20Work.pdf

General health and nutrition
- Larson Duyff, R. (2012) *American Dietetic Association Complete Food and Nutrition Guide.* Houghton Mifflin Harcourt
- http://dietsindetails.com/article_fat.html
- www.bda.uk.com
- www.caloriesecrets.net
- www.dietitians.ca
- www.eatright.org
- www.freelancedietitians.org
- www.fruitsandveggiesmorematters.org
- http://healthylivingforlife.com
- www.helpguide.org
- http://m.ibosocial.com/Shipe/pressrelease.aspx?prid=250421
- www.mayoclinic.org
- www.mikesweightlossstory.com/Whole_Grain_Foods.html
- www.nutritionblognetwork.com
- http://nutritiondata.self.com
- www.safefruitsandveggies.com
- www.whfoods.com
- http://wholegrainscouncil.org

Meals and snacks
- American Dietetic Association. (2009) Position of the American Dietetic Association: Weight Management. *Journal of the American Dietetic Association.* 109(2):330-346
- Miller, R., Benelam, B. Stanner, S.A., Buttriss J.L. (2013) Is Snacking Good or Bad for Health: An Overview. *British Nutrition Foundations Bulletin.* 38, 302–322
- http://frac.org/wp-content/uploads/2009/09/breakfastforlearning.pdf
- www.cookinglight.com/food/quick-healthy
- www.eatingwell.com
- www.rd.com/health
- www.realsimple.com
- www.schoolnutritionandfitness.com
- www.southernliving.com/food/whats-for-supper
- www.webmd.com

Parties
- www.cookinglight.com/entertaining
- www.dummies.com/how-to/content/cooking-for-crowds-for-dummies-cheat-sheet.html
- www.pinterest.com/juzt4j/recipes-to-feed-a-crowd

Physical activity
- http://eatingforperformance.com
- www.fitclick.com
- www.fitwatch.com
- www.glycemicindex.com

- www.healthstatus.com
- www.hsph.harvard.edu/nutritionsource
- www.jissn.com
- www.mayoclinic.org
- www.myfitnesspal.com
- www.nutristrategy.com/activitylist.htm
- www.scandpg.org/sports-nutrition
- www.sparkpeople.com/resource/fitness.asp
- www.webmd.com

Recipes
- http://allrecipes.com
- www.bbcgoodfood.com/recipes
- www.cookinglight.com/entertaining
- www.eatingwell.com
- www.epicurious.com
- www.food.com/recipes
- www.foodnetwork.com
- www.realsimple.com/food-recipes

Shopping
- www.fda.gov/Food/IngredientsPackagingLabeling
- www.fruttarefruitbars.com
- www.healthcastle.com/healthy_kitchen_staple.shtml
- http://salestores.com/
- www.webmd.com/food-recipes/features/healthy-ingredients
- www.yasso.com/products

Special health concerns
- Brown, J. (2011) *Nutrition Through the Life Cycle.* Wadsworth, Cengage Learning
- Christie, C. (Ed.). (2013) *Manual of Medical Nutrition Therapy.* Florida Academy of Nutrition and Dietetics
- Eckel RH, et al. *AHA/ACC guideline on lifestyle management to reduce cardiovascular risk: A report of the American College of Cardiology American/Heart Association Task Force on Practice Guidelines.* Circulation. 2013
- Go AS, et al. *Heart disease and stroke statistics—2014 update: A report from the American Heart Association.* Circulation. 2014
- Lewis, A. (2013) *Celiac Disease: Basics & Beyond.* Professional Development Resources. www.pdresources.org/course/index/1/1148/Celiac-Disease-Basics-Beyond
- Lichtenberg, M. (2006) *The Open Heart Companion: Preparation and Guidance for Open-Heart Surgery Recovery.* Open Heart Publishing
- McDonald, L. (2014) *Quick Check Food Guide for Heart Health.* Barron's Educational Series
- National Heart, Lung, and Blood Institute. (2006) *Your Guide to Lowering your Blood Pressure with DASH.* U.S. Department of Health and Human Services
- www.nhlbi.nih.gov/health/public/heart/hbp/dash/new_dash.pdf

Continued on next page

Resources
(continued)

Special health concerns

- University of Chicago Celiac Disease Center. (2013) *Jump Start your Gluten-Free Diet: Living with Celiac Coeliac Disease & Gluten Intolerance.* Gluten Free Passport
- USDHHS. (2006) *Lowering your Blood Pressure with DASH.* U.S. Department of Health and Human Services
- www.aaaai.org/home.aspx
- www.camplejeuneglobe.com/sports/article_659da148-1b09-11e3-8c44-001a4bcf887a.html
- www.cancer.org/healthy/eathealthygetactive
- www.celiaccentral.org
- www.cureceliacdisease.org/living-with-celiac/resources
- www.diabetes.org/food-and-fitness
- www.eatright.org
- www.ext.colostate.edu/pubs/foodnut
- http://fnic.nal.usda.gov/lifecycle-nutrition
- www.foodallergy.org
- www.heart.org
- www.how-to-lower-cholesterol.com
- www.mayoclinic.org
- http://mylifecheck.heart.org
- www.nhlbi.nih.gov/health/public
- www.nia.nih.gov/health/publication
- www.nlm.nih.gov
- www.nutrition.gov/life-stages/seniors
- www.wpbs.org/parents/food-and-fitness/eat-smart/stay-on-track-with-healthy-snacks
- www.sharecare.com/health/diabetes/how-dairy-diabetes-meal-plan
- www.thatsfit.com/2009/12/03/healthy-kids-snacks
- www.womenshealth.gov/publications/our-publications/fact-sheet/hashimoto-disease.html

Index

Credits

Books are a labor of love—and in this case teamwork, too. Many thanks to all the contributors, as well as Katie LeGros, who helped with preliminary edits, Pam Chally, the Dean for the Department of Nutrition and Dietetics at the University of North Florida (and the department's number one fan), and my husband, George, who forwent his loved days at the beach on weekends to stay home with me while I wrote. Thank you also to Kate Kirby and Katie Crous at Quarto.

With special thanks to Jenni Davis for writing the following articles:
• Superfoods, pages 52–55
• Unmasking marketing, pages 66–67
• 5 Ways to overcome sugar cravings, pages 108–109
• Potato chips and the alternatives, pages 120–121

Quarto would like to thank the following agencies and manufacturers for supplying images for inclusion in this book:

a9photo, Shutterstock.com, p.59cbl • Afanasieva, Olha, Shutterstock.com, pp.21b, 48bl • Africa Studio, Shutterstock.com, p.118b • All ingredients images on pp.31, 61, 81, 86b, 87b, 97t, 101t, 105t, 107, 115, 117bl, 119, 123, 127, 133b, 134b, 137t Shutterstock.com • amenic181, Shutterstock.com, p.132t • AN NGUYEN, Shutterstock.com, p.47br • Andrey_Kuzmin, Shutterstock.com, p.123br • antpkr, Shutterstock.com, p.114t • Ariwasabi, Shutterstock.com, p.37 • B. and E. Dudzinscy, Shutterstock.com, p.15 • Baibaz, Shutterstock.com, p.55b • Bain, Kitch, Shutterstock.com, p.59t • Banner, Shutterstock.com, p.54tl • Barbone, Marilyn, Shutterstock.com, p.84t • Bergfeldt, Barbro, Shutterstock.com, p.137b • Beth Galton, Inc., StockFood, p.28t • Bozhikov, Aleksandar, Shutterstock.com, p.5tl • brulove, Shutterstock.com, p.117t • Cobraphotography, Shutterstock.com, p.77 • Cooke, Colin, StockFood, p.75b • dannylim, Shutterstock.com, p.126br • Drfelice, Shutterstock.com, p.59ctl • Duncan, James, StockFood, p.73bl • Eising Studio—Food Photo &Video, StockFood, pp.2bc, 34, 121b • Elisseeva, Elena, Shutterstock.com, p.28bl • Elovich, Shutterstock.com, p.2tr • EM Arts, Shutterstock.com, p.108 • Foodfolio, StockFood, p.59b • FoodPhotogr. Eising, StockFood UK, p.85b • friis-larsen, Liv, Shutterstock.com, p.83c • Gayvoronskaya_Yana, Shutterstock.com, p.99t • Gerber, Gregory, Shutterstock.com, p.4tc • Getty Images, pp.18, 24, 45, 71, 81, 91 • goldnetz, Shutterstock.com, p.115bl • Gray, Michael C., Shutterstock.com, p.73t • Guyler, David, Shutterstock.com, p.133t • Hera, Jiri, Shutterstock.com, p.56b • Hong Vo, Shutterstock.com, p.136b • HONGYAN, JIANG, Shutterstock.com, p.17cl • Image courtesy of www.cosmed.com, p.95t • In Green, Shutterstock.com, p.129 • ISTL, StockFood, p.20 • Istochnik, Shutterstock.com, pp.134–135t • iStockphoto, pp.2tl, 14, 52tc, 66c • Jackiso, Shutterstock.com, p.2c • Jasmine_K, Shutterstock.com, p.32c • JOAT, Shutterstock.com, p.49bl • Karandaev, Evgeny, p.27br • Karandaev, Evgeny, Shutterstock.com, p.13 • Kentoh, Shutterstock.com, pp.72b, 75tr • Kesu, Shutterstock.com, p.73br • Kovac, Juraj, Shutterstock.com, p.76 • Kristensen, Lasse, Shutterstock.com, p.2cbl • Kucherova, Anna, Shutterstock.com, p.50c • Leonori, Shutterstock.com, p.2tc • M. Unal Ozmen, Shutterstock.com, p.17br • Mackenzie, Robyn, Shutterstock.com, p.84b •

Maria, Lapina, Shutterstock.com, p.32bl • Melica, Shutterstock.com, p.120 • MJ Prototype, Shutterstock.com, p.125b • Molin, Kati, Shutterstock.com, p.26bl • Mycteria, Shutterstock.com, p.2br • Narodenko, Maks, Shutterstock.com, pp.52tl/tr, 126br • Nattika, Shutterstock.com, p.126bl • Olson, Tyler, Shutterstock.com, p.65 • Omelchenko, Anna, Shutterstock.com, p.2bl • OPOLJA, Shutterstock.com, p.99b • Papp, Ildi, Shutterstock.com, p.5tr • Photo Cuisine, pp.2ctl, 3tl/bl, 5tc, 46t, 49, 51, 53, 60bl, 78, 82bl/tr, 85t, 87, 121t • Pierre Javelle, StockFood, p.54 • Piyato, Shutterstock.com, p.79b • Popova, Olga, Shutterstock.com, p.47c • pr2is, Shutterstock.com, p.97b • Razumova, Valentina, Shutterstock.com, p.3bc • Resnick, Joshua, Shutterstock.com, p.92 • Restyler, Shutterstock.com, p.23br • Sarsmis, Shutterstock.com, pp.3tc, 105b, 113 • Schild, Rena, Shutterstock.com, p.131 • Shaiith, Shutterstock.com, p.3br • Sheridan Stancliff, StockFood, p.74b • SOMMAI, Shutterstock.com, p.103br • Spaxiax, Shutterstock.com, 19br • Staroseltsev, Alex, p.3tr • stockcreations, Shutterstock.com, p.117b • tarog, Shutterstock.com, p.119t • Tepsuttinun, Winai, Shutterstock.com, p.28br • Tkacenko, Andris, Shutterstock.com, p.133cr • Topseller, Shutterstock.com, p.4tr • Viktor1, Shutterstock.com, p.17t • Vincek, Dani, Shutterstock.com, p.16b • Volkov, Valentyn, Shutterstock.com, p.59b • Volosina, Shutterstock.com, p.46b • Vostok, Dan, Shutterstock.com, p.67 • wheatley, Shutterstock.com, p.124t • Wierink, Ivonne, Shutterstock.com, p.109b • Wiktory, Shutterstock.com, p.57

All step-by-step and other images are the copyright of Quarto Publishing plc. While every effort has been made to credit contributors, Quarto would like to apologize should there have been any omissions or errors, and would be pleased to make the appropriate correction for future editions of the book.